HEALTHY MUSLIMAH

Be the best version of yourself!

By

ZOHRA SARWARI

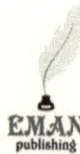

EMAN
publishing

Cover Design by Madeeha Shaikh

Printed in the United States of America

Dedication

'(Our Lord! Accept this from us; You are the All-Hearing, the All-Knowing).'

(The Qur'aan: Chapter 2, Verse 127)

TABLE OF CONTENTS

INTRODUCTION

REFUSING TO SETTLE FOR MEDIOCRE

My journey for weight loss began shortly after I got married. I thought I could eat whatever I wanted and I was immune from gaining weight. I was only nineteen, and young. Little did I know I was gaining everything I ate.

About three months after I had been married we were going to my cousin's wedding and I was so excited. However every time I tried a dress on, it didn't fit. I realized I had gained some weight. I mean, I was eating everything and I wasn't stepping on the scale nor was my husband complaining, so I assumed it must have not been much weight. I bought a pretty black dress, and I bought a girdle so that it would make me look skinnier. I had to suck in all the fat.

Well I thought I looked great that night. I walked in smiling, with my head up high. Everyone looked so much skinnier that night. Everything was going great until I ran into an aunt of mine.

She meant well, and is such a nice lady, but we have all faced family members that sometimes are a bit too upfront. So this aunt of mine looked at me and said, "My dear, congratulations! You must be pregnant?" I was shocked at what she had just said. I knew full well that I wasn't pregnant. I just smiled and walked away. That night I felt very uncomfortable. If she thought I was pregnant then what did everyone else think of me? My self-esteem fell to the floor and I wanted to hide. I didn't want to see anyone and I didn't want to take any pictures.

That was the beginning of my journey to lose weight alhamdulillaah. Within three months after that I lost about 20 pounds and looked almost my original weight. My journey for gaining and losing weight had begun.

CHAPTER ONE

MY STORY OF GAINING AND LOSING WEIGHT

Growing up in a Muslim family we are told by Allaah (Subhaanahoo wa ta'aalaa)-(God Almighty) in The Noble Qur'aan, that as women we need to cover ourselves and be modest. Our bodies are only for our husbands to see and our beauty is only for our immediate family and husband. This means that when we meet others, and communicate with others, they would only be interested in who we truly are as a person, and not what we look like.

Your inner beauty is what counts the most; your outer beauty is for those who are closest to you. It is hard to understand a concept such as this in a society where people feel the more we beautify ourselves the better, and outer beauty has taken precedence over our inner beauty.

As a Muslim I am taught that we don't judge people for what they wear or how they behave. We respect people for who they are regardless of how different they may be. Personally, I am more interested in finding out who an individual is, and not what they look like on the outside.

In the Qur'aan, God Almighty says:

"O mankind! We have created you from a single male and a female, and made you into nations and tribes, that you may know one another."

(The Qur'aan, Chapter 49, Verse 13)

It was at that moment that it struck me and made me think what I used to be thin and fit. I mean I had gained weight after marriage, but then I lost it. I wasn't happy with what I was today; I looked at myself immediately and found that I had put on weight due to neglected calorie intake, and several pregnancies. I mean I was slim, and under my modest abaayah, everyone who saw me thought I was fine. However, I knew better, I knew that I had to lose at least 20 pounds, and my body was not the shape it was after my first two children.

After six pregnancies and four kids my life became extremely busy. I barely had time to eat, forget trying to fit proper exercise in daily. I would take a walk every day, and eat healthy for the most part. I was always into health and fitness, but this last year due to so many changes I was doing it at a minimal level. Again, to many I looked fine; especially for someone who had four kids, but I knew that my expectations were higher than the normal. I am a high achiever, and I try to do my best in all that I do. I am not perfect, but if I do something, I put in all of my heart and soul.

The first thing that came to my mind was the idea that I can be an inspiration for every other woman, especially women who are mothers and those who are working. We need to take care of our bodies regardless of whether people see us or not; it is the fuel that gets us going, and allows us to be most productive. I know this, because I have gained 40-70 pounds several times in my life, including through all of my pregnancies.

My journey began 19 years ago and I have managed to lose it every time, alhamdulillaah (All praise and thanks belongs to God alone). However, I wanted more this time. I didn't want to just be slim. I wanted to be toned and have more energy, in shaa' Allaah - God Willing.

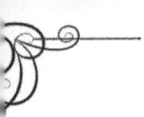

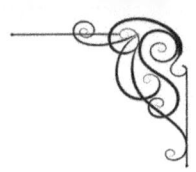

CHAPTER TWO

MY MAJOR GOALS

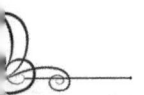

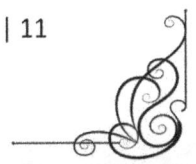

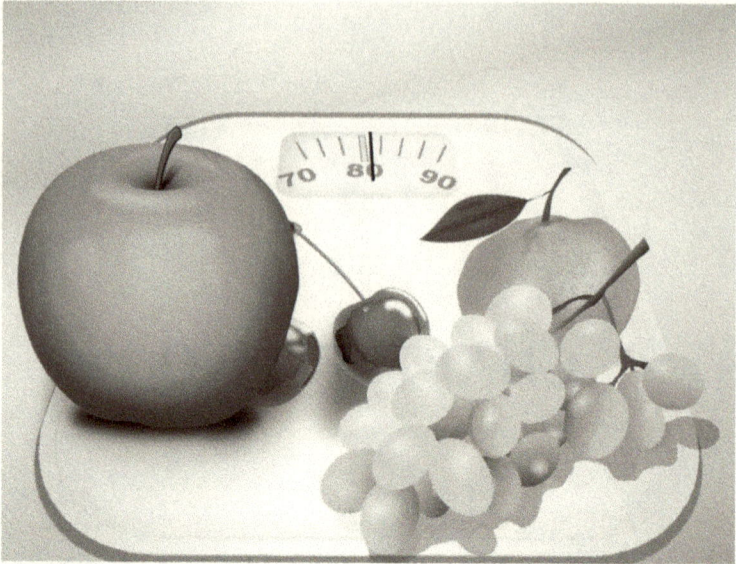

I have a very hectic daily routine. Being an author, life-coach, speaker, student of knowledge, and, most importantly, a mother and teacher to my children, is not so easy. This keeps me busy the whole day, until I am so exhausted that there is no room left for me.

Homeschooling takes the majoirty of my day. This is 6-7 days a week, and I try to balance the other duties as best as I can.

I was always a slim person before marriage, but after marriage I somewhat got a little out of shape, but recovered alhamdulillaah. However, after my third baby, and fourth pregnancy, I just kind of left the last 20 pounds that I had gained. I mean I lost about 50 pounds with my last pregnancy, but the last 20 kind of stuck around.

After my fourth child my life got so busy in dealing with four kids, business and daily routine that I just didn't care about the last 20 pounds. Since I wore modest clothing, no one else realized it as well.

In the profession that I belong to, I am working daily in triggering life-changing thoughts in other people's minds in order to help them break free from their setbacks and worries. This meant I had to practice what I preach; I needed to be in the best of health if I was to dish any advice out to others.

There were five things I really wanted to see different in me in shaa' Allaah - God Willing:

• I wanted to have more energy and be more active.

• I wanted my body fat to be 20% or less.

• I wanted to implement an exercising routine 5 days a week.

• I wanted my body to be in the best shape ever.

• I wanted to balance my life with my busy routine.

It was my first week. I began the challenge; three months to lose my last 20 pounds, and tone up. I began fasting Mondays and Thursdays for the sake of Allaah, as I needed the good deeds, and also the discipline of not eating so much.

Fasting has many benefits alhamdulillaah, yet I was unaware of them until this last year. There are 1.6 billion Muslims all over the world, so I know for a fact that many of them fast every Monday and Thursday. Little did I know how fasting would be amongst the biggest aids in helping lose weight, and eat less. My daily routine begins around 5:00 a.m. with daybreak and goes on till almost 10:00 p.m. and sometimes later.

The most difficult thing was deciding what to pre-cook, and getting the meals, snacks and lunches for the coming week ready on Saturday and Sunday to save time, as well as taking time out to exercise to remain on my commitment. Lots of scheduling was needed for this part.

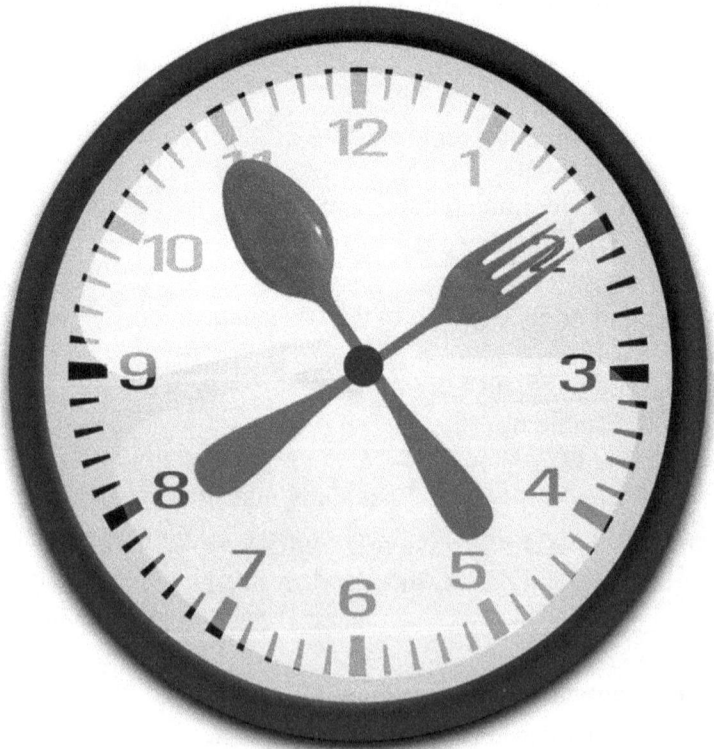

CHAPTER THREE

HOW TO EAT LESS AND LOSE WEIGHT

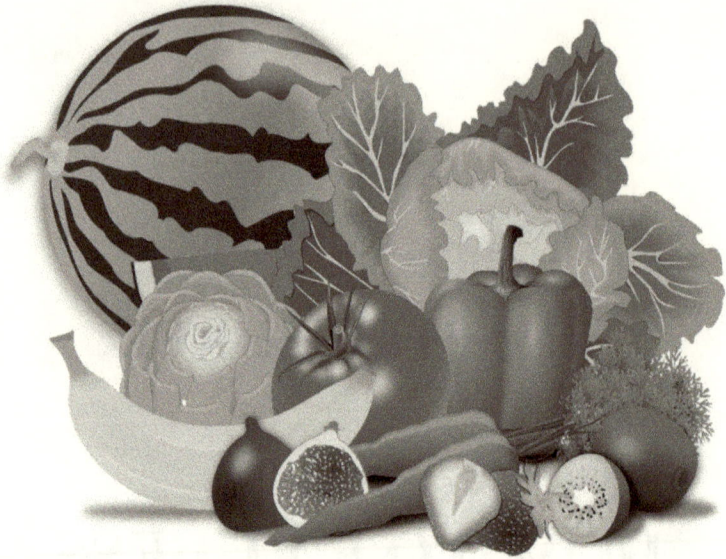

Food is a fundamental requirement for living and as such the prime objective of eating and drinking is to allow the body to function generally. The availability of food or its deficiency significantly influences the destiny of an individual. Many of us live to eat, and we overeat.

The Prophet Muhammad (peace and blessings be upon him) said; *"A human being fills no worse vessel than his stomach. It is sufficient for a human being to eat a few mouthfuls to keep his spine straight."*

(Sunan Ibn Maajah Vol. 4, Book 29, Hadith 3349)

Did you know that to lose weight eighty percent of it has to do with the foods we eat and twenty percent has to do with exercise? This means we must eat less and eat the right foods in shaa' Allaah.

Nutrition plays a big part in a life-long dieting practice. According to the divergence of cultural and geographic situations, human dietary patterns differ from one person to another. It is important to combine nutrition in the proper quantity to ensure that proper supplies of the essential nutrients are entering into the body. This results in a healthy, well-balanced diet. I am sure you have heard of this a lot. However, I want you to read this book with an open mind, and ask Allaah to make it easy for you to make the changes you need to make, so that you can be a healthy Muslimah as well, in shaa' Allaah.

All of our meals should be combined with healthy carbohydrates, vitamins, minerals and fiber. The composition of diversified food within a meal is strongly recommended for good health. When we can't stop eating, and over eat, the excessive weight becomes the reason that many diseases enter into our bodies. At this point we start rushing to the doctors. If that isn't bad enough, on the other extreme end, sometimes we exercise without eating even the minimum requirements that our bodies need. Exercising while fasting provides instant results on the outside; however, on the inside it can cause severe, internal damage.

What we eat is essential, however, even healthy food can stop us from losing weight if we eat too much of it. I don't recommend excessive calorie restraint, but there are a number of tips you can utilize to slightly decrease the quantity of food you eat, without feeling deprived. I will show you some simple guidelines to keep your body healthy, in shaa' Allaah. Remember you only have one

body; so take care of it the best that you can in shaa'
Allaah.

How To Eat Less And Still Have Energy?

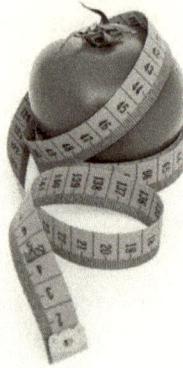

Oftentimes when I mention we need to eat less, I get
looks of shock and horror. "What? How will I function? I
will have no energy. I will faint."

*"O men, eat the lawful and good things from what is in the
earth."*

(The Qur'aan, Chapter 2, Verse 168)

The Almighty has commanded us to eat everything from
this universe, provided that those foods are lawful (halaal),
good quality (tayyib) and obviously obtained rightfully. In
reality it is statiscally stated that the majority of us eat more
than our fair share. We pile our plates up with delicious
food. We may need only half of it to fill us up, but we eat

all of it. This leads us to gain weight, have pain and in some cases suffer from illnesses. See, we are aware of this issue that we have, we know what consequences we may face if we don't change our eating habits, yet very often we cannot restrict ourselves.

Science tells us that a balanced diet and proper eating habits can facilitate weight loss and improve our energy levels. It is only through a balanced diet that we may receive energy; because a balanced diet supplies essential vitamins and nutrients to the body which are needed to metabolize everything. Let's learn about the foods which you can consume less of and yet they provide you with more energy.

Sometimes people take different dietary programs for rapid weight loss; some start fasting everyday, others quit one type of food or another, and others take pills and medications to help them. This can cause complications such as anemia, uneasiness, giddiness, etc. It is important not to stop eating to reduce weight but to make better choices of what types of food to eat in shaa' Allaah. Those foods include:

1.   Fiber-rich breads and oatmeal,

2.   Lean proteins like white meat chicken,

3.   Beans and nuts,

4.   Fish,

5.   Fruits; oranges and bananas, raspberries, blueberries, strawberries,

6.   Vegetables; all green vegetables, carrots and peppers,

7.   Dairy; milk, yogurt and low fat cheese.

Foods to avoid are those made with sugars and carbohydrates such as white candy, pastas/breads, baked goods and sodas; because these foods will result in weight gain and loss of energy.

Now, if an individual asks to prescribe a formula to lose weight and preserve energy I will suggest the following guidelines:

a)   To eat a variety of high-energy, high-value foods, but less of it.

b)   To take foods that contain moderate calories and to set a plan to have 1,200 to 1,800 calories per day.

c)   To restrict fat intake to not more than 30 percent.

d)   To make a habit of eating fiber-containing food/fruits.

e)   To avoid processed foods, and limit it to not more than eight times in a month.

f)   To limit the intake of soda and sweets.

Finally, I recommend when you're not fasting on Mondays and Thursdays to eat every few hours. If you have a menu written down then you will eat what is on it. A banana for a snack, carrots with lunch, and salad with dinner are all good items to have on your menu. This will keep you fresh, energized and healthy. Remember our stomach is similar to the fuel tank of a vehicle; if that tank is kept at its fullest, the fuel will spill out of the top. If your stomach is filled to the top, you will feel drowsy because your body will start using the preserved energy to digest the food.

The Qur'aan advises the same thing,

"Eat and drink and be not excessive"

(The Qur'aan, Chapter 7, Verse 31)

CHAPTER FOUR

THE BASICS OF WEIGHT LOSS

The Basics of Weight Loss

The basic principle of losing weight is about burning more calories than what you eat. This seems to be very simple; but if we could have internalized this simple theory there would not be any overweight or underweight problems in the world. The reality is completely different; we cannot burn more calories than we consume. So as a result we launch drastic actions like crash diets, pills or peculiar fitness devices to see direct results that promise instant achievement, but sustain it only for a short time. Very soon we regain the lost weight plus some. The true secret to weight loss is to formulate small but lasting changes in your life in shaa' Allaah.

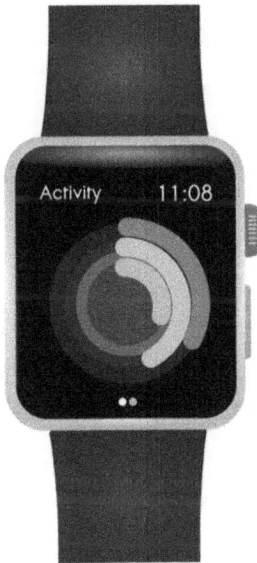

The Rules of Weight Loss

In order to lose one pound of fat one must burn approximately 3500 calories. This might be frustrating, and you are probably wondering how it is possible to burn so many calories? Well don't give up! If you follow my guidelines and proceed according to my step by step process, in shaa' Allaah, you will definitely be able to burn or cut out those extra calories. If you are adamant to lose weight, follow the following steps:

a. Evaluate Your BMR (Basal Metabolic Rate): BMR is the consumption of calories that your body wants to maintain for the smooth execution of basic bodily functions like breathing and digesting. This is the smallest amount of calories that you have to consume each day. It has to be remembered that no calculator will be 100% error free, so you should adjust these numbers as you are aware of your own metabolism.

b. Estimate Your Activity Level: Maintain a daily and weekly activity diary and use a calorie calculator to find out how many calories you burn throughout the day while standing, sitting, exercising, lifting weights, etc. At the end of the day and week, find out the average of burned calories, and then assess the daily and weekly calorie burning rate. One of the things that I recommend to do is to buy an Activity Tracker and wear it on your wrist. This has helped me and many others out there to stay on track of our goals maa shaa' Allaah tabaarakAllaah. You can buy them from Amazon.com or any retail store close by.

c. Be Conscious of Each of Your Meal Calories Consumption: Keep a sharp look at your meal calories consumption and write down what you eat and drink daily. At the end of the week find out the total calories consumption and plan accordingly on how to burn all those extra ones.

d. Make a Summary: Get your BMR number and add your activity calories. From that total subtract your food calories. Then come to a conclusion; if you are eating more than your BMR + your activity calories, you are at risk of gaining weight.

Suppose Layla's BMR is 1500 calories and she could burn 800 calories through regular exercise, morning walking and doing household works. To maintain her weight, she needs to eat 2300 calories (1500 + 800= 2300). However, according to her food journal, Layla finds that she is eating 2600 calories per day. This means that Layla will gain more than one pound within the next 2-3 weeks due to the consumption of an additional 300 calories.

The Ideal Rate of Weight Loss

The ideal rate of weight loss should be 0.5-2 pounds per week but it varies from person to person and depends on each individual's physical condition. However, a standard and a well-experimented weight loss chart is given below:

The Ideal Rate of Weight Loss Based VS. How Much Fat You Need To Lose	
Amount Of Fat To Lose	Ideal Rate Of Weight Loss
Above Average (Considered amount of more than 100lbs fat to lose)	2lbs (or more) per week.
Average (Considered amount of more than 30lbs fat to lose)	1-2lbs per week.
Below Average (Considered amount of 10lbs or less fat to lose)	0.5-1lb per week.

Managing Calorie Intake For Weight Loss

The physicians and doctors have a standard scale to assess weight in comparison to the BMI. The scale is given below:

BMI	Physical state
18.5 to 25	Healthy.
More than 25	Overweight
Over 30	Obese
Over 40	Morbidly obese

There are two basic things you must know to find out your BMI. That is your weight in kilograms and height in meters. Let us measure a BMI:

a)   Multiply your height by itself (Say 1.7 x 1.7= 2.89)

b)   Divide your weight (Say 80kg) by this figure

         (80 ÷ 2.89= 27.7)

c)   So your BMI is 27.7

Work on the habit of eating less. I have several suggestions to help you do that as well:

a)   Drink water, instead of sodas or drinks that are loaded with sugar.

b)   Eat a lesser amount of lunch than normal.

c)   Avoid sugar in tea and coffee.

d)   Take less portions of the food that you enjoy.

e)   Avoid having a second plateful at dinner.

f)   Cut out sweets, sugared biscuits and chips between meals.

CHAPTER FIVE

PRINCIPLES OF EATING FOR WEIGHT LOSS

"When I first reverted to Islaam I was exercising and young.

I went into the understanding that no men could see me work out or ride a bike. I was in a very old community of Muslims. I tried my best to stay fit but slowly gained weight. I then had my children back to back, alhamdulillaah. I tried to slim down in between but it did not happen. Before I realized I was 200 lbs, not able to do much, always tired and feeling very sad about everything.

I was also in a very oppressive marriage that did not help. I gained even more weight and before I knew it I was at a whopping 215 lbs.

My body was aching all the time, my clothing was not fitting and I was having to shop in the "BIG" girl stores. Let me say here that it is different if this is your genetic make-up, for me it was not. I was always fit and around the 8-10 dress size.

I was falling into deeper and deeper sadness.

I got a divorce and had to deal with all of the emotion that comes with that.

I so desperately wanted to play with my children outside at the park, run and kick the ball; but I was not able to. My doctor told me I was borderline diabetic.

I was in pain all of the time. I did not want to move and just barely made it to work and events for my children. I always showed a happy face but was really so disappointed with myself. What had become of me?

That is when I decided to take matters into my own hands. I cut out all complex carbohydrates. I limited any sweets. Took milk out of my coffee and was very mindful of my entire intake of carbs, milk products and sweets. I started with 5,000 steps a day, joined the gym and increased my water intake, 8-10 glasses a day.

For the gym I committed to go at the minimum 3 days a week. Max 5 days. Giving me days off; 3 days on, 1 day off, and then 2 days, and 1 day off. I did a routine of 20 minutes for cardio and then 11 flights on the stair machine and light-weights for arms. 3 – 5 sets of 10 sit-ups with 30 second pauses in between.

Now after 3 months I am up to 30 minutes cardio, 15 flights of stairs and 75 sit ups and 35 lbs – 60 lbs on arms and back.

I am now down to 167 lbs. I am active. I spend my days always active, cleaning, playing with the children, extra curricular activities, full time work and fun on the weekend.

May Allaah bless all of us to be healthy in order to live our lives here to the best of our potential - Aameen."

PRINCIPLES OF EATING FOR WEIGHT LOSS

The Five Laws of Careful Eating

The Almighty has created our body with a centrally controlled mechanism and an automatic guidance system. Our brain can signal us when we are hungry and when we are full. But it is observed that during eating we are often busy with some other job like driving, working on a computer or even watching TV, which hinders the control system to transmit the signal in time not to eat, or if it transmits the signal it cannot reach its area of operation. However, if we can follow some rules for careful eating, it is guaranteed that we will lose weight and be able to maintain a sound, healthy weight in shaa' Allaah. It is vital for our success that we maintain our healthy lifestyle for as long as we are alive.

The Five Laws of Careful Eating are:

a)   **Laws of Sitting:** When you want to eat, sit down and concentrate yourself on eating. Strictly avoid eating either standing up or while walking.

'Umar bin Abu Salamah (May Allaah be pleased with him) reported that the Messenger of Allaah (Peace and Blessings Be Upon Him), said to me,

"Mention Allaah's name (i.e., say Bismillaah before starting eating), eat with your right hand, and eat from what is near you."

(Bukhaari & Muslim)

b) **Laws of Consciousness:** There is no doubt that you are a super genius and you are capable of multi-tasking, but during eating, never divert yourself from the concentration of eating. During eating, do not break your concentration from eating; allow the body signals to alert you when you are full.

c) **Laws of Extracting Taste from Each Bite:** Always be careful with what you are eating, perceive the quality of the food and taste its flavors. Really monitor what your nerves are expressing about these foods. Experience the sensation of the food, and drink. Allow the flavors to excite your senses.

d) **Laws of a Single Bite:** Complete the chewing and swallowing of one mouthful food prior to taking another bite. Keep the fork down during this stage and eat slowly.

e) **Laws of Withdrawal:** Be relaxed while eating and enjoy the total eating environment. Always remember a stress-free eating environment can facilitate a comfortable digestion.

Nine Simple Ways Of Escaping Overeating

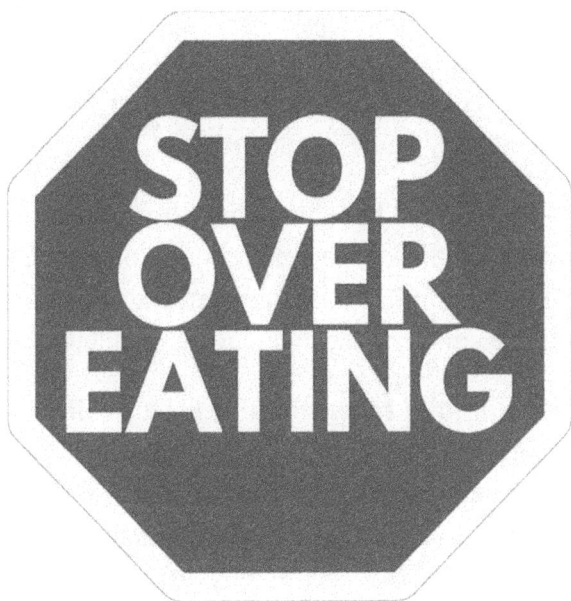

Eating is essential but Islaam advises us to not be extravagant.

Miqdam ibn Ma'd reported: The Messenger of Allaah, peace and blessings be upon him, said,

"The son of Adam cannot fill a vessel worse than his stomach, as it is enough for him to take a few bites to straighten his back. If he cannot do it, then he may fill it with a third of his food, a third of his drink, and a third of his breath."

Sunan al-Tirmidhī 2380

I will now share nine flexible tips on how to eat less.

a)   **Eating in a mini-plate:** Full plates indicate that you are eating a complete feast and a slightly full plate looks like an inadequate meal, irrespective of the actual amount of food. The similar quantity of food seems to be huge on a mini size plate. Utilization of a mini plate for escaping food is proved as one of the best methods for eating less.

b)   **Taking 20% less food in the plate:** From experience we eat 80% of the total food in one go and take another 20% to be full. So it is recommended to take 80% of the food in a smaller plate and leave 20% intentionally.

c)   **Drinking in a taller glass:** Like a smaller amount of food seems to be more food on a smaller plate, tallness makes things appear larger than size, even when the capacity is the same. A straight up column looks longer than a horizontal row; accordingly tall glasses appear superior to wide ones. You can very well discard your liquid calories consumption by choosing taller glasses rather than smaller or fatter ones.

d)   **Include protein in your breakfast:** Generally people are found to think that breakfast is a miracle weight loss cure, however, only breakfasts high in protein have been proven to lessen hunger and decrease eating all through the day.

e)   **Make a habit of eating three times a day:** It is better to eat three small meals a day, and two snacks, than to eat three large meals alone. Your body will burn the calories faster this way, in shaa' Allaah. Remember eat only when you are supposed to.

**f)	Keep munchies out of site:** Experiments have proven that the human body wants to have a lot more food when the food is in sight. To avoid additional food, store tempting foods out of sight, or better yet, out of the surroundings.

**g)	Chew persistently:** Give more attention to chewing your food. It has been observed that many people don't chew their food properly. If you are one of those who chew the least number of times before shoveling in another fork full, there is a chance that you will be eating substantially more at every meal in comparison to the thoroughly chewing peers.

**h)	Avoid eating from the package offer:** It is human tendency to have comparatively more if the price is less. Sometimes restaurants launch package offers to have a buffet dinner at a fixed price. Normally a person eats more than usual at times like this, which brings about some digestion issues and other problems.

**i)	Avoid eating in front of the TV or computer:** Normally it is our habit that we intend to have our dinner, especially our holiday meals, in front of the TV or computer, whilst watching something. As a result a vast majority of people diverted eating to overeating.

"Seven Essential Foods For Weight Loss" that you should eat:

a)   **Eggs:** An egg contains a good amount of protein and gives its consumers a sense of satiety. For this reason, you will not feel hungry for a long time. This will allow you to eat less food accordingly. Naturally, you will end up with weight loss in sha' Allaah.

b)   **Lentils:** Lentils preserve an increased content of soluble fiber and protein. Both of these two nutrients have a direct effect of stabilizing the blood sugar. Increasing of fat caused by the rising of insulin secretion can be controlled by eating lentils. It's likely to prevent the fat on the abdomen especially.

c)   **Cabbage:** Cabbage is full of iron and calcium. It contains a small amount of calories and plenty of fiber, which plays a vital role in weight loss. Spinach can also be chosen as a good replacement for cabbage.

d)   **Oats:** Oats contain carbohydrates of a unique quality and a kind of very healthy food. Oats do not have any effect on blood sugar levels and give the consumers the sense of satisfaction. So it definitely plays a fundamental role in weight loss.

e)   **Chinese Wolfberry:** Chinese wolfberry preserves 18 sorts of protein, little amount of calories and is rich in beta-carotene. It is widely known as one of the best sources of protein. A tablespoon of Chinese wolfberry can control your hunger for a long time.

f)   **Salmon:** Salmon fish contains a copious amount of 3 fatty acids and improves the sensitivity of insulin. It works actively for the development of muscles and reduces the fat on the abdomen.

g)   **Apples:**   Apples contain antioxidants and a high content of pectin and fiber; which leads to a great sense of fullness. It has been tested by many that eating an apple a day can restrict weight-gain.

CHAPTER SIX

LIFESTYLE IDEOLOGY TO LOSE WEIGHT

How To Eat Less And Be Full

It is easier said than done. After all, if losing weight was simple, thirty percent of the population would not be overweight. In order to lose weight, you have to eat less and when you eat less you usually feel hungry, which most of us discover is unpleasant. That is where it falls apart for a lot of people. Nowadays, there are a number of tips to guide you on how to eat smaller amount of calories without the sense of hunger.

It is not about a diet that you eat and then fall off. It is about getting your body's appetite-controlling mechanisms working in favor of you instead of against you. These tactics can help you to lose weight and keep your bodyweight balanced in shaa' Allaah.

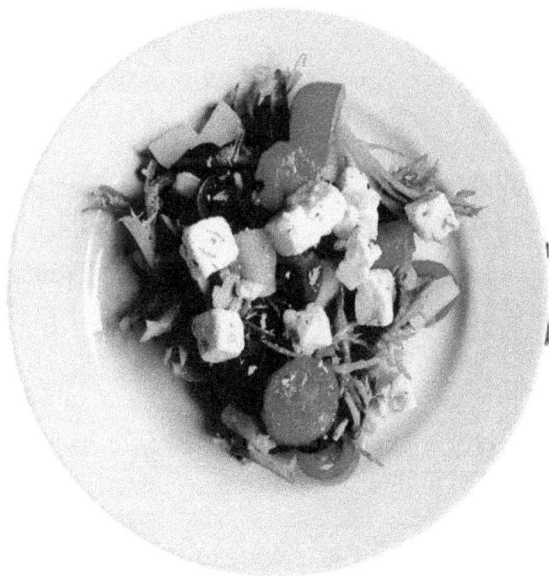

Three Tactics To Trick Your Stomach

Our stomach is as tiny as a water balloon. When it is empty, it seems to be relatively diminutive and slack. But when you fill it up, it extends and gets bigger. There are unique nerve cells in the lining of our stomach called proprioceptors that sense this stretching and send a message to our brain that the stomach is full. All of them are acquainted with the mechanism that something is filling our stomach. I will share with you three tactics that will help trick your stomach; making it believe that it is full.

First: Eat highly water content foods. Water has no calories but it occupies a lot of volume in the stomach, and that gives recognition to your proprioceptors and creates a feeling of fullness. Recently, a research analyzed that people who drank two glasses of water before meals had the feeling of being full. You can apply the same tactic by choosing foods that have higher water content over those with less water.

For example, the only dissimilarity between grapes and raisins is that a grape contains about six times as much water in them. That water makes a big difference in how much they fill you up. Ingredients of salad like lettuce, cucumbers, and tomatoes also contain very high water content. If you initiate your meals with a salad or soup, you are most likely to consume fewer calories at those meals.

Second: Grow a habit of eating foods containing a lot of fiber. The more rapidly your food is transformed into glucose and absorbed into the bloodstream, the more rapidly you will be feeling hungry. The other way to feel full on a smaller amount of calories is to select foods that are full of fiber. Like water, fiber adds volume to foods without adding calories and that additional bulk assists to fill up your stomach. That is particularly accurate when you eat fiber and fluids together, because the fiber soaks up water. Fiber has a couple of other actions; it slows down the rate at which food leaves your stomach, so that feeling of fullness exists a bit longer. Then, when the food travels into the intestine for digestion, fiber stimulates the release of a hormone called cholecystokinin, which fires another indication back to the brain along with the information that the stomach is full.

Foods that are full of fiber comprise dried beans, bran, vegetables, and whole grains. A high fiber cereal will keep you full longer than a low fiber cereal. At lunch, a cup of black bean or split pea soup will go further than a cup of cream of mushroom.

Third: Changing a little amount of the starches with protein. Another way of regulating your hunger is by looking at how swiftly your blood sugar climbs and falls after meals. That is the more rapidly your food is converted into glucose and absorbed into the bloodstream; the more rapidly you will be feeling hungry again. Carbohydrates are turned into glucose much more rapidly than proteins and fats, which need a lot more digestive steps to change. Research always demonstrates that dieters who eat smaller amount of carbohydrates and more protein are not as hungry as those who eat a higher percentage of carbohydrates.

As an example, instead of a sandwich consisting of two slices of bread and a slice of halal turkey, have an open-faced sandwich with one slice of bread and two slices of halal turkey. Both sandwiches contain about the same amount of calories but the higher protein version will keep you pleased for longer. At breakfast, you could have an additional egg and one fewer piece of toast.

How Much Exercise Do I Need?

Physical exercise is one of the best tools for weight loss, but obviously it varies from person to person. A weekly 250 minutes exercise and five days in a week ensures effective results for the human body. It is important to start small at the beginning and increase it gradually. For example with 3 days of cardio for 20-30 minutes and steadily increasing time each week, will allow your body a bit of time to adapt to the exercises.

How Much Energy Do You Need?

It is commonly observed that the tennis players are eating bananas during the match and footballers are eating oranges at half time. That means there are some diets recommended by the physicians and nutritionists to eat before the exercise, during, and at the end of the exercise, to keep good health or to minimize the risk of illness or overtiring. It is the carbohydrates, proteins and fats which provide energy for exercise. If you don't have enough energized diet for your body, you will definitely feel weak and tired, your muscles and bones will weaken suddenly and you increase risk of illness and injury.

How Many Calories You Should Eat Before Exercising

The performance of exercise is solely vested upon the diets you take before the exercise. Ideally it is important to take a small meal at least two to four hours prior to the exercise. This will energize your muscle glycogen levels. Normally glycogen acts as a fuel to have the best endurance. Nutritionists recommend eating those foods which contain adequate amount of protein to help with recovery after exercise and a high amount of carbohydrates to increase blood glucose. Some ideal meals and snacks which have been proven as the best pre-exercise meals and post exercise snacks are:

Ideal Pre-exercise meals	Ideal Pre-exercise snacks
Sandwich filled with chicken	Bananas (ripe)
Pasta with tomato-based sauce and vegetables	Smoothie made with low-fat milk
Baked beans on toast	Cereal or energy bar
Porridge made with low-fat milk	Diluted squash (not sugar-free)

If you are planning to exercise for more than 90 minutes, you are advised to ask your doctor.

How To Eat Less At Family Dinners

Eating is essential but Islaam advises us to not be extravagant. The hadeeth of the Prophet Muhammad (Peace Be Upon Him) emphasizes to eat without filling the stomach. Now the question remains, how to eat less at family events? I suggest that you sit with your family members for dinner as guided in Islaam, say "Bismillaah" (In The Name of Allaah) and start eating. Try your best to eat less.

Research has analyzed that people who drink two glasses of water before meals have feelings of being full even before starting their meals. You can choose foods that have higher water content over those with less water. As such, before dinner you may start with two glasses of water or you may serve vegetable soup ten minutes before the dinner. You will definitely find that you and your family members are eating less at dinner.

Why Most People Eat Less During Summers

The secret to weight loss is to select healthy foods and take lesser amounts of calories than you actually burn. It's easier to make lighter foods during summer; when heavy, high-calorie dishes look less appealing. Another great benefit of the summer is that during summers most people are out of the kitchen.

During the hot summer, the human body accumulates a huge amount of heat which cannot be expelled out.

When the surface temperature rises to 35 degree celsius, the human body sweats a lot which increases the magnitude of blood and compels the human body to be irritable. Being in this state, people prefer to have liquids, and as a result the amount of eating during summer lessens.

Best Summer Foods For Weight Loss

"Enjoy fresh produce in season. You will be thrilled at how fresh, delicious, and satisfying it tastes," says Susan Moores, RD, a St. Paul, Minn., Nutrition Consultant.

She also added that, *"Save the oranges and apples for fall, and load up on fresh berries, melons, greens, tomatoes, zucchini, cucumbers, beets, pea pods, and all the super-nutritious and low-calorie fruits, greens and vegetables that grow in the garden this time of the year."* The distinct method to trim calories from the summer diet is to load up on seasonal nature's gifts. There are so many delicious fruits and vegetables which are readily available at farmers' markets and in the local grocery. If you include all those summer fruits and vegetables in your daily meals it will help to reduce weight. The nutritionists usually recommend eating some of these foods to help with weight loss during the summer. They are as follows:

a)   **Children's Soups:** *"Research shows that a low-calorie, broth-based soup at the beginning of the meal will* *fill you so you eat less at the meal,"* Moores says. She advises of children's soups like gazpacho or cucumber-dill, which preserves a lot of vegetables, which helps to keep a tiptop body during summer.

b)   Watermelon: It contains 50% of water and works wonderfully to reduce weight and is considered one of the best foods during the summer.

c)   Grilled Vegetables: Nutritionists strongly recommend grilled vegetables as the best food for summer. It is the composition of grilled onions, bell peppers, zucchini, carrots, eggplant, asparagus, and garlic.

d)   Fruit-Based Desserts: Nutritionists also suggest including fruit-based desserts, as it helps to lose weight. She recommends the dessert composition should be grilled banana sundaes with low-fat ice cream, frozen grapes, grilled white peaches with blackberries and honey, etc. Moores says *"Just give the produce a quick rinse; slice, dice, toss fruits, vegetables, low-fat cheese, a handful of toasted nuts with some salad greens and a light raspberry or ginger vinaigrette, along with a whole-grain roll, and you have a meal in minutes."*

CHAPTER SEVEN

MOTIVATION FOR EATING LESS

How To Motivate Yourself To Eat Less

"O Children of Adam! Look to your adornment at every place of worship, and eat and drink but waste not by extravagance, certainly He (Allaah) likes not those who waste by extravagance."

(The Qur'aan: Chapter 7, Verse 31)

The Qur'aan strongly discourages overeating and encourages a balanced diet; Allaah condemns everyone who is extravagant, even in things that are permissible.

One of the main principals of good health is a balanced diet. Good foods must contain nutrition, benefit and capability of producing required energy; it must be light for the stomach in order to enable easy digestion. If all those qualities are absent in any kind of food, it is obvious that these foods must be avoided. It is better to have a balanced diet which is less in amount instead of overeating. The Prophet Muhammad (Peace Be Upon Him) emphasized the habit of eating less as a means of preventing sickness and diseases. Overeating is the root of almost all the complexity that we have today.

Prophet Muhammad (Peace Be Upon Him) is reported to have said:

"The son of Aadam does not fill any vessel worse than his stomach. It is sufficient for the son of Aadam to eat a few

morsels to keep him alive. If he must fill it, then one-third for his food, one-third for his drink, and one-third for air."

(Tirmidhi – declared saheeh by al-Albaani)

The Prophet (Peace Be Upon Him) said,

"A believer eats in one intestine (is satisfied with a little food), and a kaafir (unbeliever) or a hypocrite eats in seven intestines (eats too much)."

(Bukhaari)

If anyone eats too much, he becomes sluggish and sleeps a great deal, and wastes a lot of his time.

Sufyaan al-Thawri said that, *"If you want your body to be healthy and to sleep less, then eat less."*

It was said that eating too much also makes the heart hard and heedless of Allaah.

Ibrahim Ibn Adham said:

"Anyone who controls his stomach is in control of his deen, and anyone who controls his hunger is in control of good behavior. Disobedience towards Allaah is nearest to a person who is satiated with a full stomach, and furthest away from a person who is hungry."

The Ulamaa' enumerate multiple benefits of eating in moderation. Eating less keeps the body healthy and light, keeps the heart soft, increases memory, weakens desires, and disciplines the soul, while excessive eating brings about the opposite of these praiseworthy qualities.

Haatim al-Taa'iy said in Fath al-Baari that, *"If you give your stomach and your private part what they ask for, you will end up regretting it."*

We must be motivated to eat less as The Qur'aan and Hadith advise us to eat less. A Muslim believes his food and drink is a means to something else. They are not an objective and pleasure in themselves. The Muslim eats and drinks in order to keep his body healthy, so that he may worship Allaah, the Almighty. This is the worship that will make us qualified for the honor of the life and happiness of the Hereafter. We do not eat and drink for the sake of eating and drinking itself or its desires. Therefore, if we are not hungry, we do not eat. If we are not thirsty, we do not drink.

Eating Less In Light Of Islaam

A mother is seldom found in this world not forcing her kids to eat; to finish their plates until they are full. We also do the same for ourselves. What we don't appreciate is that this is not only bad for our health, but it is also against the judicious teachings of our beloved Prophet (Peace Be Upon Him). It is this excessive eating that is keeping us far from the honest and focused devotion of Allaah and the peace that should be there in all our worship. The reason is that overeating makes the body heavy, which leads to being sluggish in our devotion. All of us can address from our experiences in Ramadhaan, when the devotion of Allaah becomes profound and painstaking, if we had too much to eat.

'Umar (May Allaah be Pleased With Him) said: "By Allaah, if I wanted I could wear the finest clothes among you, and eat the best food, and have the most luxurious life. But I heard that Allaah will condemn people for some of their actions and said:

'You received your good things in the life of the world, and you took your pleasure therein. Now this Day you shall be recompensed with a torment of humiliation, because you were arrogant in the land without a right, and because you used to rebel against Allaah's Command (disobey Allaah).'"

(The Qur'aan; Chapter 46, Verse 20)

Not only is overeating unhealthy for the physical condition of an individual, it is equally bad, rather worse, for his spiritual health and happiness, as well as for his aakhirah.

Ibn 'Umar said: A man burped in the presence of the Prophet (blessings and peace of Allaah be upon him) and he said:

"Keep your burps away from us, for the one who eats his fill the most in this world will be hungry for the longest time on the Day of Resurrection."

(It was also classed as hasan by al-Albaani in Saheeh at-Tirmidhi)

The wisdom behind whatever the Prophet Muhammad (Peace Be Upon Him) said or did 1400 years ago is being proven now with science, and it shows the truthfulness of his Prophethood and the beauty and excellence of our Deen, al-Islaam, the perfect way of life.

The way to stop eating too much is to stop gradually. If an individual is used to eating a lot and he stops all of a sudden and starts eating very little, he will become weak and his hunger will increase. So he should reduce it steadily, by eating less and less of his usual food, until he reaches a moderate intake of food, in shaa' Allaah.

When it comes to eating better, Islaam recommends less is definitely more. Besides, eating less is the perfect way to lose those extra pounds we have been trying to discard for years. We forgot that the paramount and most perfect diet is to follow the Sunnah of the Prophet Muhammad (Peace Be Upon Him). Indeed, it is only his way that is the best and his guidance that is perfect.

What Is The One-Third Rule?

Prophet Muhammad (Peace Be Upon Him) is reported to have said:

"Nothing is worse than a person who fills his stomach. It should be enough for the son of Aadam to have a few bites to satisfy his hunger. If he wishes more, it should be: one-third for his food, one-third for his liquids, and one-third

for his breath."

(Tirmidhi, Ibn Maajah and al-Haakim)

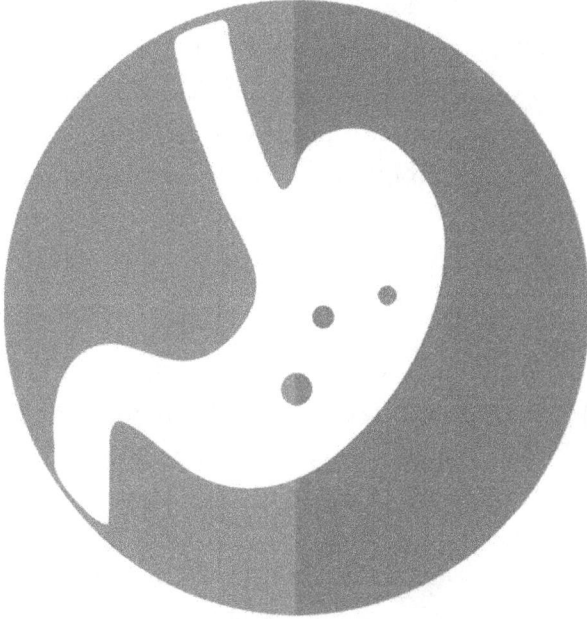

This is called the one-third rule for eating less in light of Islaam. The Prophetic guidance on the best of common diets is: "one third food, one third water and one third air." Once the stomach is saturated with food, it will have insufficient place for water. When the food and water both exceed the exact level of the stomach, that individual will feel heaviness of the body, pulmonary difficulties, excessive stress, exhaustion, and insufficient supply of oxygen and blood to the lungs. For good health, nutritionists and medical science also recommend to follow the one-third rule.

The Secret Two-Third Dieting Rule

The 'two-third' dieting rule and eating-strategy are planned to be very simple to realize and follow. You are given enough freedom for more than one-third of the time. Your dieting habits will modify for the better, and your overall physical condition will develop. The famous eating strategy and secret 'two-third' rule narrates that you must be particularly careful about your physical condition, and what you make your mind up to swallow at least two-thirds of the time, 5 days a week. At these times you eat all that you think is good.

The nutritionists suggest that breakfast and lunch each should be one-third, leaving two-thirds for the rest of the day. It is advised to carry this out 5 days a week. This means that you are going to do the whole thing that you consider healthy for two of the three meals daily. Ultimately you will do this 7 days a week. Remember this is not a diet; this is a modification of your eating-style. Motivation is the key for this to work. You can identify what is healthy, and what is not! Just hold on to what you know is healthy when you eat. Your brain will begin to think in a healthy way, which leads to a life that will become instinctive, and this will become natural eventually in shaa' Allaah.

Drinking fresh juice is a great way to go in the morning. Also, grab a banana, yogurt, and a handful of nuts on your way out of the door. Think healthy all the way up until dinner time. I suggest you have a handful of nuts 45 minutes before the dinner. You will not be as hungry, and have a preference to eat less. If you pay attention to this rule, you will obtain the results that you are looking for. It has worked for so many people maa shaa' Allaah. I assure that with the eating-strategy of the 'two-third' eating rule, you will lose weight and feel great in shaa' Allaah. Also don't forget to always make du'aa for your success.

The 2 & 5 Rule!

According to the nutritionists, the human body should consume at least 2 servings of fruit and 5 servings of vegetables on a daily basis. This is considered part of a healthy diet. As research has revealed a lifestyle that incorporates sufficient amounts of fruit and vegetables can help prevent and lessen the exposure of developing cancer, constipation, obesity, heart diseases, high blood pressure and high cholesterol. It is thus enormously significant that one eat ample amounts of vegetables and fruits to make sure that one's body is receiving the nutrients that are required on a daily basis.

In Australia, researchers have revealed that the common adult only eats 2-3 servings of vegetables per day (half of what is recommended) and 1-2 servings of fruit per day. This indicates that on average, lots of people should still try and increase their daily fruit and vegetable intake in order to confirm that their body is getting its optional nutritional requests.

However, the key motive why the average person consumes half of the recommended daily consumption of fruit and vegetables, and why many people discover it is hard to follow this rule, is that eating 2 servings of fruit and

5 servings of vegetables means that you have to eat a lot. An example of a serving is described below.

a)   Nutrition values of one serving of fruit:

One dish up of fruit is equivalent to:	1 piece of fruit including apples, oranges and bananas, or;
	15 grapes, or;
	6 strawberries, or;
	½ cup of freshly squeezed juice

b)   Nutrition values of one serving of vegetable:

One dish up of vegetable is equal to:	½ a cup of cooked vegetables
	1 whole tomato
	10 baby carrots
	1 cup of salad vegetables

Thus, theoretically, you would have to eat 2 pieces of apples, 3 cups of salad vegetables, 10 baby carrots and another full cup of cooked vegetables in order to achieve the 2 & 5 rule; and we have not even taken protein and carbohydrates into consideration yet.

Still, controversy exists; how can we make sure that we are eating the right amount of fruit and vegetables to achieve our best possible nutritional requirements? A few ideas to help you reach your goals are listed below:

1)   If you don't like to eat fruit, drink a mug of your preferred squeezed juice during breakfast. It is your every day suggested serving of fruit taken care of.

2)   In the place of day snack, eat baby carrots with low-fat dip such as hummus.

3) Maintain healthy guidelines that incorporate more fruits and vegetables in it.

4) Make sure that you always include vegetables in your lunch and dinner. For lunch, an excellent proposal is to include tomatoes, beetroot and onions in your sandwich, and have a bowl of fresh salad and light dressing on the side. For dinner, always add a sald before your meal. If you are stir-frying, add vegetables such as capsicum, onions, beans and bean sprouts.

5) If it still seems to be tough to consume the everyday suggested intake of fruit and vegetables for a healthier body, vitamins can be consumed if necessary.

Remember, becoming healthier requires a lifestyle change. Even if you are adding supplements, by no means can you supplement an unhealthy diet. Eating healthier and developing a healthy diet is still fundamental for a healthy lifestyle. If your current diet needs changing, start with small changes and set yourself goals. This will make sure that you remain and continue your enthusiasm for a healthier body.

CHAPTER EIGHT

RAPID WEIGHT LOSS TRICKS

"It's been a year and half since I started college, and approximately a year since my weight began to gain up on me. The experience in itself wasn't one I felt entirely worried by, because there was always the naïve feeling that some way, I was going to shed everything in due time.

Unfortunately, by the end of my first year in college, I realized that wouldn't be the case. I came to realize I had added just about enough weight to get my entire being solely focused on how I look. I used to be a perfect size 4, but now I had gone to a size 12.

Time felt like it stood still and my pain only magnified as my cravings for unhealthy food consumed me, while my clothing became impossible to fit me anymore. Losing the fit I once shared with my clothes didn't stop there, as my confidence took a major hit when my friends, decided they couldn't cope with having to walk with someone who didn't care to take care of themselves.

The feeling of "loneliness" crept in slowly, joined by its companion "depression" and "disgust" for my own body. Days passed by into months, and my confidence, morale, and will to carry on through life waned desperately and dangerously and I recalled times without count where going out suddenly became a thing I was most dreadful of.

My social life slowly cared away as well and all I could enjoy was the "me time" with the only pair of friends still willing to indulge a "fatso" like me; my pizza deliveries and chicken wings.

My life had slowly gone from being one filled with optimism to one where I second-guessed my existence on every turn and wondered if the following day could ever be brighter for me. I cried to no end and struggled in every aspect of my life until the realization that the only one who could help me through my situation was Allaah. I began praying again and making lots of du'aa. I needed to change myself in order to get Allaah's help. I remembered the aayat where Allaah says in Surah Ar-Ra'd in Aayat 11: "Allaah will not change the condition of a people until they change what is in themselves."

So, I decided to buckle up and start working out. I altered my diet and began to eat well and appropriately without eating the dangerous fats and carbs which weren't helping my body or health. The journey seemed incredibly long and tiring and I came close to giving up on every turn but the determination not to become an object of ridicule by those around me and those who didn't know me but would make jest of me on first contact, drove me forward.

Months passed and the progress was slow, but my heart had begun to find some warmth of joy again. It slowly began to heal and my mental strength dragged itself from the stage of depression and sad thoughts back into one of strength and belief over the next few months. My body healed from the damage caused to it by my obesity and my confidence took a shot of strength well needed for me to begin to enjoy life again. I was very thankful to Allaah for His help and for blessing me with strength to do it.

No less than six months after I began intense workout and dieting, I had lost 30 lbs, and realized the joy in having friends again as I made new friends built towards helping me remaining in shape and in the right frame of mind. It ended up being the best feeling of freedom mixed with joy and gratefulness as the days went by.

I want to let you all know that no matter what stage in life you are and this happens to you, to not give up. Believe in yourself, and then believe that Allaah will be there to help you, you just need to ask Him."

RAPID WEIGHT LOSS TRICKS

There are several weight loss tricks that can help you lose fat quickly and easily, in shaa' Allaah. I have already mentioned some tips, but I want to make sure that you get them ingrained in you. I will repeat some of them and also give you some new ones.

Despite the numerous ways to lose weight and eat well many individuals suffer from weight problems. However, there are many, many ways to slim down rapidly. As many a diet plan has stated (when describing the competition), "Rapid weight loss tricks the body into thinking you're starving and overwhelming you with hunger." Generally, for each deficit of 3,500 calories you create, you are going to lose a pound of excess fat.

You can find various rapid weight loss tricks that can help in reducing your weight easily. To get fit and lose weight quickly this appears to be one of the primary goals of our modern society. Almost everyone will say it's about good diet and nutrition. However, the number of people with weight problems is growing constantly. Although slimming down in only a few weeks is certainly possible, usually it will take at least a couple of months. While losing weight quickly is difficult, its not impossible either. If you have the appropriate attitude and knowledge it is possible to achieve excellent results, in shaa' Allaah.

In order to slim down effectively, you will have to work very hard and need a good plan. You diet, you lose fat, you gain weight, you diet, you slim down...and so it goes on. In order to shed weight faster, one of the best rapid weight loss tricks is to just eat less and exercise considerably more.

To keep reducing your weight you will have to consume a well-balanced diet that includes a variety of foods. Slimming down too quickly can have a negative effect on your central nervous system and may cause you to feel sluggish and drained. When you drop a lot of weight quickly, you are losing water mainly and muscle, instead of body fat. Losing around 1 to 2 pounds weekly is smart and healthy. In adjusting your diet plan, one way to lose fat is with antioxidant and mineral rich, Cacao Chip Nuggets. Weight loss workouts will also allow you to slim down a lot faster. Drinking water will help you feel full and this can be helpful to shed weight. By eliminating calories every day you will lose those pounds and keep them off permanently. Alhamdulillaah by the mercy of Allaah, I was able to shed weight and maintain it while not having to turn to pills or other extreme measures. Excellent well-balanced meals and exercise is all you need to have great results.

Use this eighteen evidence-based keys for successful weight management. You don't have to follow all of them, but the more of them you apply into your life, the more likely you will be successful at losing weight. The more this becomes habit, the easier it will be in keeping the weight off longterm. Consider adding a new step or two every week or so, but keep in mind that not all these suggestions work for everyone. That is, you should pick and choose those that feel right for you to customize your own weight-control plan. Note also that this is not a "diet" per se, and that there are no forbidden foods.

1.   Start With a Healthy Diet: That means a diet that's rich in vegetables, fruits, whole grains, and legumes, and low in refined grains, sugary foods, and saturated fats. You can include fish, poultry, and other lean meats, and dairy foods (low-fat are preferable to save calories). Aim for 20 to 35 grams of fiber a day from plant foods, since fiber helps fill you up and slows absorption of carbohydrates.

2.   Keep an Eye on Portions: You can eat all the broccoli and spinach you want, but for higher-calorie foods, portion control is the key. Check serving sizes on food labels, some relatively small packages contain more than one serving, so you have to double or triple the calories, fat, and sugar if you plan to eat the whole thing. Popular "100-calorie" food packages do the portion controlling for you (though they won't help much if you eat several packages at once).

3.   Eat Mindfully: This involves increasing your awareness about when and how much to eat using internal (rather than visual or other external) cues to guide you. Eating mindfully means giving full attention to what you eat, savoring each bite, acknowledging what you like and don't like, and not eating when distracted (such as whilst watching TV, working on the computer, or driving). Such an approach will help you eat less overall, while you enjoy your food more. Research suggests that the more mindful you are, the less likely you are to overeat in response to external cues, such as food ads, 24/7 food availability, and super-sized portions.

4.   Eat Slowly, And Chew Well: A component of mindful eating, this allows more time for satiety signals to reach the brain (it takes about 20 minutes), so slow eaters tend to feel more full and eat less. The process of chewing itself may also stimulate hunger signals. In addition, eating slowly makes you more aware of the smell, taste, and texture of the foods, which can lead to greater satisfaction with fewer calories. Keep in mind also that the most pleasure often comes from the first few bites of food; after that, it's the law of diminishing returns. Thus, you should focus on those first few tastes of chocolate, cake, or other indulgences, as this may be enough to satisfy.

5.   Don't Rely on Willpower: Instead, control your "food environment" so that you don't unconsciously overfill your plate and eat when you are not hungry. That means, for example, not having junk foods at home or at least keeping them out of sight (such as on a top shelf or in the back of the fridge), and changing your routine; so you don't regularly encounter temptations (such as avoiding the office pantry between meals if it has enticing foods and driving a route that doesn't take you past your favorite food places). This helped me a lot, alhamdulillaah. By not having the sweets in the home, I wasn't able to eat them.

Use smaller plates, bowls, cups, and utensils when you eat and drink in shaa' Allaah. You may even want to invest in portion-controlled plates (that delineate what reasonable serving sizes are) or portion-control devices (that allow you to measure your food directly on the plate); many different kinds are available online.

Portion out snacks into small bowls or bags; don't eat from large bags or boxes. You may not have control over everything in your food environment, but being aware of hidden food triggers and traps may be enough to keep you from overeating.

6.   **Identify Emotional Triggers (that may be making you overeat):** For example, you may eat more when you are stressed, depressed, upset, angry, lonely, or even happy and excited. To distinguish between real hunger and emotional eating, rate your hunger/fullness levels before, during, and after eating on a scale of 1 to 10, with 1 being "beyond hungry" or "starving" (with associated headaches, lightheadedness, and weakness) and 10 being "beyond full" (as in after-Eid-meal stuffed). Ideally you should eat when you are at level 3 (hungry but not yet uncomfortable) and stop at level 7 (full and satisfied). If you often eat for reasons other than hunger, find pleasurable non-food-related activities that you can do instead, such as going for a brisk walk or run.

7.   **Go for Volume (low-energy-dense foods):** Eating foods low in energy density that is, with fewer calories relative to their weight and volume increases satiety, so you are likely to fill up on fewer calories. This well-tested concept was first developed by Barbara Rolls, PhD, at Pennsylvania State University in her well-regarded Volumetrics eating plan. In general, the best way to lower the energy density of your diet is to eat more foods that have a high water and high fiber content (notably fruits, vegetables, broth-based soups, and cooked whole grains), in place of low-moisture or high-fat foods (such as cheese, crackers, cookies, and fried potatoes). Incorporate more of these foods in recipes, add more vegetables to soups, stews, and pasta dishes. For example, fill sandwiches and wraps with lots of lettuce, chopped cucumbers, and grated carrots; top whole grain pizzas with more vegetables and less cheese. Snack on popcorn and grapes instead of raisins (for the same 120 calories, you can eat more than a cup of grapes compared to only 1/4 cup of raisins).

8.   **Get Adequate Protein (and include some with all meals):** There's evidence that protein increases satiety more than carbohydrates do. Protein also helps limit muscle loss during weight loss. Look for sources of lean protein (such as beans and other legumes, white-meat poultry, and low-fat or non-fat dairy) or those also rich in healthy fats (such as fish, nuts, and soy foods). Some research suggests that distributing your protein throughout the day also helps in weight loss rather than eating the bulk of it at, say, dinnertime.

According to a 2015 paper in the American Journal of Clinical Nutrition, higher-protein diets that include at least 25 grams of protein at each meal may reduce appetite and thus body weight, compared with lower-protein diets. However, people with or at high risk for kidney disease, and that includes many older people, should be careful not to consume excessive amounts of protein.

9.   Eat Regularly (don't skip meals) and Choose Healthy Low-Calorie Snacks: Many people find that going longer than a few hours without food makes them more likely to overeat later (often on high-calorie treats). Find a meal-timing pattern that works best for you. If you eat between meals, plan ahead for healthy "mini-snacks" (100 to 200 calories), such as a small container of low-fat yogurt with a handful of berries; two tablespoons of hummus with a cup of baby carrots or sliced bell peppers; a slice of cheese or two thin slices of turkey on half a whole-grain pita; an ounce (small handful) of nuts; or a tablespoon of peanut butter and a banana.

10.   Limit Variety at Meals: Variety in your overall diet is important to ensure that you get a range of nutrients and other substances that contribute to good health; but having too many choices at once can lead to overconsumption (the "smorgasbord effect"). This is because foods with different flavors and sensory qualities whet the appetite, even if you are physically satiated— which is why there always seems to be "room for dessert." It's also easier to overfill your plate when you have a large number of choices. On the other hand, you're likely to eat less if you have less variety, since foods similar in taste and texture dull the palate (a phenomenon called sensation-specific satiety). Be especially careful at all-you-can-eat buffets and parties. Scan the whole array of foods before making your selection; choose no more than three or four items that appeal to you most, and make only one trip. Using smaller plates also helps limit your choices.

11.   Don't Drink Your Calories: Beverages are not as satiating as solid foods, and people usually do not compensate for liquid calories by eating less food. It is okay to drink milk but otherwise stick with water or other non-caloric beverages like tea and coffee (watch the cream and sugar). Choose whole fruits over juice. What about diet beverages? The jury is still out on whether they help with weight loss. The proposed 2015 U.S. Dietary Guidelines do not recommend sugar substitutes, citing a lack of evidence that they help in long-term weight loss. To liven up water, try a squeeze of lemon or lime or other fruit essence.

12.   Cook at Home Often: That allows you to eat more whole foods and control how much oil, sugar, and other high-calorie ingredients you use. Studies have shown that people tend to eat more when they eat out, though you must still be careful to limit portion sizes at home. If cooking from recipes, look for healthy lower-calorie ones that include nutrition analysis, and stick to the serving sizes. Be aware also that just as restaurant portions have ballooned in recent years, recipe serving sizes have also been on the increase.

13.   When Eating Out, Follow these Simple Rules: Take advantage of calorie listings on menus (or online beforehand) to find lower-calorie options. Don't order anything that's been super-sized, and consider sharing entrées (or asking for half to be wrapped to take home before you start eating), or have an appetizer or salad as your main dish.

Reading over the whole menu before you order and asking questions of your server or the chef can help steer you towards more healthier, lower-calorie options.

Request that dishes be prepared with no or minimal butter, oil, or other high-fat ingredients, and ask for salad dressings on the side, so you can control how much you use. And be aware of the menu "tricks" that restaurants use to boost sales often of cheaper and less-healthier foods. I do this often by going to the website of the restaurant and looking for the nutrition facts. After I read the calories and fat in each item, I make an executive decision on what is best for me to eat. The calories and fat change my mind from unhealthy to heathier foods. Alhamdulillaah.

14.   Allow for (Controlled) Indulgences: Most people find foods high in fat and sugar pleasurable, since they activate the body's "reward system" (which releases chemicals in the nervous system relating to pleasure). Overly restricting such foods (or any other types of food you crave) can be counterproductive, since it can increase your desire for them and lead to bingeing. An occasional treat is fine, as long as it doesn't tip the scale with calories. You might, for instance, have a small daily treat or save up for some treats on weekends. On the other hand, some people can't eat just a little and may be better off avoiding hard-to-resist foods altogether.

15.   Keep a Food Diary: Studies, including one in the Journal of the Academy of Nutrition and Dietetics, have found that dieters who regularly record what they eat lose more weight than those who don't. It doesn't matter how you do it; in a notebook, on the computer, or with an app on your phone, as long as you record your intake consistently and honestly (including even condiments and tastings you may take while cooking). This simple act makes you more accountable for what you eat and helps you see patterns in your eating habits that may be contributing to weight gain.

16.   Get Enough Sleep: An often overlooked factor in body weight may be your sleeping habits. Though the optimal amount of sleep varies from person to person, too little sleep (fewer than six hours a night in one study) has been linked to weight gain because it may affect appetite hormones and lead to increased hunger and food intake, decreased calorie burning, and increased fat storage.

17.   Consider Weighing Yourself Regularly at Least Once a Week: This increases self-awareness and can provide encouragement if the numbers are going in the right direction or it can motivate you to get back on track if you detect an upward trend. A 2014 study of 40 overweight people found that more frequent self weigh-ins were associated with greater weight loss and that going more than a week without stepping on the scale was associated with weight gain. Regular self-weighing is a particularly effective strategy for maintaining long-term weight loss, according to the National Weight Control Registry, which tracks people who have successfully lost and kept weight off. However, whether you weigh yourself and how frequently you do it, is a personal decision. Some people get discouraged by small fluctuations that occur over the course of a day or several days (which reflect normal shifts in fluid levels, rather than changes in body fat). Keep in mind also that weight is not everything: another good, and sometimes better gauge of weight loss success is to measure your waist and other body areas, such as your hips and thighs.

18. Set Realistic Goals and Have a Realistic Body Image: Just as weight tends to creep up over time, shedding excess pounds takes time. Don't expect to be able to lose 10 pounds a week (any diet that says you can is counting on water losses, not fat loss). Small and steady losses; about one to two pounds a week usually win the race in the long term. For most people, losing just 5 to 10 percent of body weight will provide health benefits. Also keep in mind that depending on your body type and genetics, you may never be able to get back to your high school or college weight. And if you and your family members tend to have a certain body shape (like a pear, for example), weight loss will result in overall slimming but won't reshape your body.

CHAPTER NINE

NUTRITIONAL EATING PLAN FOR WEIGHT LOSS

MEAL PLANS – IMPORTANT

I would like you to stick to the meal plan as best as you can. If there is something on the menu that you don't like, then please select something else from the meal plan to eat. Note: It is okay to eat the same meal twice.

Example: Quinoa, seeds and nuts, replaced by porridge and berries. The foods chosen on this plan give you a wide variety of different meals to eat throughout the week in shaa' Allaah. Trying new foods and meals helps maintain a balanced eating plan, as all foods provide different nutrients to help maintain a healthy lifestyle.

Ten Important Points

1. You will have to take some time to think about food preparation. We all have time; we just need to make it. Most of us leave the house on a daily basis and hope that we can buy food from the shops, which tends to be unhealthy. Most of the time it's quick, convenient and full of hidden ingredients which aren't great for our health or our waist lines. Always look for the best options of food choices if you are caught leaving the house without your own food.

2. It is 28 days, not 28 years. This is a great period of time to change. Please remember this if you are struggling after the first week. Results at the end will be worth it. You will always experience

difficulty when you make a change; stick with it and you will feel great after.

3. When going to a social event it is not hard to stick to the plan. You can still have a glass of soda, eat meats and vegetables etc. You may be surprised how accommodating people can be.

4. It won't be easy… most things in life which are worth achieving are not. As you continue throughout the process, things will become easier.

5. Ignore the doubters. People, who can't do things themselves, often try and drag people down with them. Ignore them, stay on track and let your results speak for themselves.

6. Please remember the basic rule of calories in versus calories out. Not all calories are equal, but eating a whole bag of nuts because it says eat high levels of fat will still encourage weight gain. Think about portion control. The advantage of this plan is it increases satiety, which leads to people eating less.

7. Do not underestimate the power of water. Often we are thirsty, not hungry. Drink lots of water, not diet coke or orange squash water. Increasing your trips to the toilet is worth the trade-off for great results.

8. Try to do your best to follow the plan. If you fall off the wagon and eat junk food, don't stress about it. Check your plan and get back to eating proper food. This isn't an all or nothing plan. One mistake doesn't make you unhealthy.

9. Please forget all of the conventional wisdom that you have been educated with over the last 40 years, i.e. that fat makes us fat; it's bad for our heart and health. We have eaten good sources of fats for thousands of years. There is no clear evidence on how eating good sources of fat is bad for our health. It has only been during the last 40 years that we have reduced our fat consumption (even olive oil, butter) and the average person now weighs 20 lbs more than they did in the 70's. This is quite sad when we think about it. This is a discussion for another time but the key statement to remember is that FAT does not make you FAT.

10. This plan is encouraged to make you aware of healthy food choices, improve your energy levels and make you feel great. The by-product of eating well and feeding your body with healthy, nutritious food is you will also lose weight. Don't become obsessed with the scales.

WEIGHT LOSS SAMPLE MEAL PLAN (Women)

MEAL PLAN	DAY 1	DAY 2	DAY 3	DAY 4	DAY 5	DAY 6	DAY 7
BREAKFAST	BREAKFAST	BREAKFAST	BREAKFAST	BREAKFAST	BREAKFAST	BREAKFAST	BREAKFAST
						SMOOTHIE (Mix all ingredients below together in a blender)	
1 Protein Unit	1/2 cup fat free vanilla yoghurt	175ml fat free milk	175ml Fat Free Yoghurt	1 Boiled Egg, with Grilled Tomato	30g grated low fat cheese	1/4 cup fat free Yoghurt & 1/4 cup Fat Free Milk	40g Grilled Kipper, with grilled tomatoes & mushrooms
1 Starch Unit	1/2 cup All bran or Hi-Fibre bran	¼ cup oats cooked in the fat free milk	1/2 cup Swiss-style muesli	1 slice Rye bread or seed loaf, Toasted	1 low GI bran muffin	2 Tbs. oat-bran	1 slice low GI bread, toasted
1 Fruit Unit	1 Tbsp. raisins	1 sliced Banana	5 Sliced Strawberries, added to cereal	1/2 cup Freshly Squeezed Orange Juice	1 small banana	1 small Banana & 80g Mango	1/2 small mango
1 Fat Unit	1 Tbsp. flaked almonds	2 tsp. peanut butter, added to porridge	1/2 Tbsp. flaked almonds	2 tsp. peanut butter	(fat in muffin)	1 Tbsp. flaked almonds	2 tsp. peanut butter
SNACK	SNACK	SNACK	SNACK	SNACK	SNACK	SNACK	SNACK
1 Fruit Unit	1 Yellow Cling Peach	3-4 Strips Dried Mango (30g)	1 Large Apple	4 slices fresh Pineapple	1 Pear	1 Cup Fruit Salad (140g)	A handful of grapes
LUNCH	LUNCH	LUNCH	LUNCH	LUNCH	LUNCH	LUNCH	LUNCH
1 Protein Unit	1 TBSP Fat Reduced Hummus & 20g (2-3 slices) Shaved Turkey	2 Chicken Strips	30g Smoked Salmon	30g Beef Strips	1/2 tin of tuna or salmon	30g Clover low fat cheese	2 mini Chicken Kebabs (40g)
1 Starch Unit	1 slice Low GI Seed Bread	2 mini Pita Breads, lightly toasted	1 slice seed bread	1 small cooked Mealy	1/2 cup cooked pasta	3 Provitas or 2 Ryvitas	1 cup cubed sweet potato, to roast
WITH Vegetables	Rocket, Lettuce, Sliced Tomatoes, Cucumber & Spring Onions	Fill pita with fresh coriander, cherry tomatoes and sweet Peppers	Butter Lettuce, Cherry Tomatoes, Pickled Cucumbers, Sprouts & Snap Peas	Shredded Coleslaw, grated Carrots & Diced Cucumber	Lettuce, rocket, diced Carrots & Grated Beetroot	Butter lettuce, Rosa Tomatoes, Orange Peppers & sliced Onion Rings	Roasted Vegetables: diced Pumpkin, Brinjals, Sweet Peppers, Mange tout Peas, Onion & Garlic

	DAY 1	DAY 2	DAY 3	DAY 4	DAY 5	DAY 6	DAY 7
Other	Lemon Juice	Raspberry Vinegar for dressing	Fresh lemon Juice for Dressing	Cranberry Balsamic Reduction	Lemon juice	Pickled onions or gherkins	Fresh herbs
1 Fat Unit	1/4 Avocado	1 Tbsp. Low Oil Mayonnaise	1/4 Avocado or 2 tsp. Seed Mix	1/4 Avocado Pear	2 tsp. low oil mayonnaise	1 TBSP Low Oil Dressing	1 tsp. Olive oil for Roasted Vegetables
AFTERNOON SNACK	SNACK	SNACK	SNACK	SNACK	SNACK	SNACK	SNACK
1 Dairy unit	175ml fat free yoghurt	175ml milk with 3 tsp. Milo	2 low fat cheese wedges	175ml milk with coffee	175ml fat free yoghurt	1/2 cup fat free cottage cheese	175ml milk with 3 tsp. Milo
1 Fruit Unit	1/2 Medium Mango	1 Pear	2 Kiwi Fruit	1/2 Large Grapefruit	150g Paw Paw	3-4 Provitas	1/2 cup Fresh Fruit Juice
DINNER	DINNER	DINNER	DINNER	DINNER	DINNER	DINNER	DINNER
3 Protein Units	Skinless Chicken Breast (90-100g) - marinated and grilled or braaied	100g Grilled Hake, with Basil Pesto & Cherry Tomatoes	120g Beef strips & Vegetable Stir-fry	120g Grilled Salmon	120g pork fillet medallions marinated in orange juice	100g beef steak - grilled or braaied	120g Grilled Ostrich fillet
Free Vegetables	Beetroot and Carrot Salad with raspberry vinegar for dressing	Roast Vegetables (Sweet Peppers, Butternut, Cauliflower, Baby Marrows, Onions, Garlic)	Stir-fry Vegetables	Steamed Asparagus, with Fresh Lemon Juice & Olive Oil; & Carrot Salad	Large mushrooms & Gem Squash	Raw Baby Spinach Leaves, Sundried Tomatoes, grated Carrots, Spring Onion	Baby lettuce leaves, rocket, baby corn, mange tout, peppers with balsamic reduction
1 Fat Unit	1/4 avocado	Basil Pesto	1 tsp. Olive oil in cooking	1 tsp. Olive Oil	1 tsp. Olive oil in cooking	1 Tbsp. Low Oil Dressing	1 tsp. Olive oil in cooking
EVENING SNACK	EVENING SNACK	EVENING SNACK	EVENING SNACK	EVENING SNACK	EVENING SNACK	EVENING SNACK	EVENING SNACK
1 Fruit Unit	1 cup Mixed Berries	1/2 tin Sliced Peaches in Natural Juice	4 slices fresh pineapple - can be added to stir-fry	2 Dried Pear Halves	1 Banana	1 wedge watermelon	200g sliced Strawberries

125 ml = ½ cup

250 ml = 1 cup

375 ml = 1 ½ cups

WORKPLACE DIET TRAPS

We spend on average about a third of our day at work, so we should really think about what we are eating there as well. All too often our workload, stress, tiredness, lack of time and temptation combine to derail our best intentions. With a bit of planning, you can use snacks and lunch to keep your diet on track, your energy levels up, and even save a bit of money.

Here are some tips to make workplace eating healthier for you:

Eat breakfast

A healthier breakfast will set you up for the day and stop you becoming hungry before lunch in shaa' Allaah. If you're not hungry before leaving home, have breakfast at work.

Bring Your Own

Home-cooked food is often lower in calories and fat, and cheaper than food bought on the high street. If sandwiches aren't your thing, you could cook extra in the evenings and take the leftovers to work; saving you money.

Drink Water

Drinking water regularly may help keep hunger pangs in check. You should aim to drink about six to eight glasses (1.2 litres) of fluid every day.

Plan Your Snacks

Keep healthier snacks within reach, such as fruit, vegetables (e.g. carrot sticks and reduced-fat hummus dip) or homemade popcorn (without fat, sugar or salt).

Swap Crisps

If you have a bag of crisps at lunch, go for oven-baked crisps, which can contain up to 70% less fat than regular crisps, or a plain rice cake.

Go Lean

Instead of fatty meats such as halaal sausages, go for lean meats, such as turkey or chicken, tuna and salmon or even a hard-boiled egg. Remember to go easy on the mayo!

FOOD CRAVINGS

However good our intentions, when a food craving strikes it can be a real test of our willpower. There is debate about why we have cravings; they can be caused by our emotions and by such things as stress, boredom, habit or insecurity. Use these tricks to help combat cravings:

Don't Go Hungry

Hunger can make cravings worse. Keep your energy levels topped up with some healthier high-fiber snacks.

Drink Water

Some people fnd water helps to calm cravings; because water is filling, it can trick your body into thinking it is satisfed. Hot drinks have the same effect.

Find a Distraction

Find an activity to take your mind off your craving; go for a walk, have a bath, call a friend, or listen to some Qur'aan.

Chew Some Gum

Some people find chewing sugar-free gum curbs their appetite; but don't overdo it as chewing more than 20 sticks of gum over a day can make you ill.

Brush Your Teeth

Brush your teeth with toothpaste. Once your mouth is minty clean and fresh, some people find it helps to get rid of a craving.

Reduce Temptation

You are less likely to crave unhealthy foods if they are not readily available – so avoid buying them!

Set a Time Limit

Cravings are fleeting. Try holding off for 30 minutes and fnd something to distract you in the meantime. Chances are, your urge will pass once the time is up.

Have a Small Portion

If the desire just won't go away, give in, but do it the smart way: have a small portion and reduce your calorie intake later to stay on track.

THINK BEFORE YOU DRINK

Drinks from lattes to colas can also lead your calorie count to creep up. What you drink should not be overlooked when trying to lose weight. Drinking too many sugar-sweetened drinks can contribute to weight gain.

So what are the common offenders and where could you be going wrong?

Coffee:

Getting a caffeine fix could give you 193 cal or more in one hit if you opt for cappuccino or mocha. Switch to black or white coffee instead.

Fruit juice and smoothies:

You might feel virtuous guzzling these but watch out. A small glass of cranberry or apple juice racks up nearly 100 cal and a small 250 ml yoghurt based smoothie can be about 136 cal. Go for fruit-only smoothies instead. Although fruit juice counts towards your 5 A DAY, you may find eating pieces of fruit more filling.

Soda:

Lemonade or cola is not only bad for our teeth but it adds an additional 140 calories by drinking just one can. It is best to drink it once in a while and opt for diet soda.

CHAPTER TEN

EXERCISE FOR BUSY MOMS

It is no wonder with all that mothers have to do, that sometimes busy moms tend to gain weight or have a hard time still losing the past baby weight that they have gained. Whether the mom works outside the home or is a stay at home mother, it can be difficult to find time to workout. Most busy moms just want to sit down for 5 minutes and rest when they can, but what they don't realize is that regular workouts can actually help them have more energy for their day.

At-home workouts are the best options for busy moms. They don't have to worry about taking the time out of their already packed schedules to drive back and forth to a gym or recreation center. Instead they can simply sneak away to another room for a few minutes to get some exercise in.

We all know how difficult it is to stay in shape and find time to exercise - especially for women with babies or small kids. There's the sleep-deprivation factor, no time and priority changes. So what are the fitness options for busy moms?

The fact is, the more you take care of yourself and the better you feel, the stronger you will be physically and emotionally to take on the day with the "little ones" and all of life's challenges.

Below are some quick, but effective, exercises - specifically designed for the busy mom - for the back and shoulders to keep you strong and prevent future injuries that may occur with poor lifting and poor posture. The heavy weight of not just the baby, but also all the fun gadgets you are expected to lug around. It is no surprise that our bodies need a little help to get through the day.

Lunges

The move: Keeping your shoulders back and your eyes looking forward. Step your right leg forward. Lower your hips, creating a 90-degree angle bend in both of your knees.

Your front knee should be directly above your ankle and neither knee should touch the floor. Bring your hips back up to return to the starting position. Put your other foot forward and repeat.

Be sure to engage your core as you complete each lunge.

When to squeeze it in: You can complete this exercise in the middle of cooking dinner (stationary lunges) or making a trip to the waste basket, mailbox or street corner (moving lunges).

Arm Curls

The move: Hold onto an object, such as a bag of groceries or full water bottle, and drop your arm down to your side. Make sure your palm is facing forward holding the item.

Use your bicep muscle to pull the object upwards towards your shoulder. Slowly bring your hand and the object back down. Complete a set of 5 or 10 on each side.

When to squeeze it in: Perfect for bringing groceries to the car or in the midst of cooking, you can tone your arms while completing other chores. Just pull something out of your cupboard to act as arm weights.

Crunches

The move: Lay down on your back, with your knees bent and your feet flat on the floor. You can place your hands behind your head with the elbows out to the sides, or put your hand in front of you. Whichever one is more comfortable for you. Then lift yourself from the floor towards your knees. Your head, neck and shoulder blades must lift off the floor. When you reach by your knees hold it for two seconds, then slowly go back down and repeat it again. Complete a set of 30 crunches.

When to squeeze it in: When your kids are playing on the floor, be next to them and do this exercise. It is so easy: and you can keep the focus on them.

Squats

The move: Stand upright and move your feet to be shoulder-width apart. Begin sitting backwards, keeping your knees from sliding forward. Continue downwards until you are unable, or when you are in a nearly 90-degree angle position. Keep your back straight during the exercise.

When to squeeze it in: Complete a set of 5 or 10 squats whenever you have a break between work meetings, playing with your child or putting in a load of laundry. You can even do a few squats with your baby in arms or while picking up toys.

Tricep Dips

The move: Find a piece of furniture like a chair or couch. Firmly plant your feet on the ground about shoulder width apart with your back to the piece of furniture. Hold yourself up using your hands on the furniture.

Walk your feet out so that your legs are nearly straight. Begin dipping your hips towards the ground, creating a bend in your arms. You should feel a flex of your tricep muscles. Push yourself back up slowly using your tricep muscles. Continue for a set of 10 tricep dips.

When to squeeze it in: During a news show or break from cleaning the house, complete a set of dips. This move will help tone your arms and gain added muscle strength.

By adding in exercises into the small moments of your day, you can maintain a healthy, active lifestyle without needing to go to the gym or take time away from your family.

EXERCISE MOTIVATION

When you start a new exercise regime it is normal to experience some soreness. Muscles you didn't even know you had are giving you grief and it may all feel like a bit of an uphill struggle. And it's not just your body; one of the biggest barriers to getting into an exercise routine is your mind. We are creatures of habit, and if you have not done much for a while, fnding the motiovation to get up and go can be a real mental battle. But don't be discouraged. You are going through the beginner's pain barrier and after a week or two, this should be a distant memory.

If you feel your enthusiasm dipping at any point, here are our top 10 tips to boost your motivation:

- ✓ Be realistic. Remind yourself that you want to become more active because it will help you become healthier and lose weight. It is a crucial component of your journey.

- ✓ Schedule it. Plan your exercise at the start of the week and put it in your diary. Planning in advance when, how and where you will exercise will increase your chances of making physical activity a normal part of your lifestyle. Even simple approaches like laying out your running kit or packing your gym bag the night before can help.

- ✓ Pat yourself on the back. Look back at your weekly food and activity chart to remind yourself how much you have already achieved.

- ✓ Don't share your plans and achievements with other people; you don't want to get 'ayn or hasad.

- ✓ Phone a friend. Find a friend or a relative to exercise with, or perhaps join a group or club. A workout buddy can provide feedback, support and entertainment – they also put pressure on you to turn up!

- ✓ Pump yourself up. Listen to a good lecture while you exercise.

- ✓ Be flexible. Change activities if you are not enjoying them. If cycling isn't doing it for you, why not go jogging or even try some fitness classes at the women's gym instead.

- ✓ Remember, the hardest part of exercising is getting out of the door – so once you have passed that hurdle, it should be plain sailing.

- ✓ Set goals. They don't need to be grand achievements. For instance, try to walk a little bit more each day, take the stairs instead of the lift or walk part of the way to work. Keeping a written record of these mini-goals can help you to see your progress over time.

✓ Reward yourself. Set yourself non-food rewards for achieving stages along the way. There's nothing like an incentive to spur you on.

CHAPTER ELEVEN

COMMON MISTAKES PEOPLE MAKE WHEN TRYING TO LOSE WEIGHT

"I have an awesome husband! But one thing that he had a problem with was his addiction…to soft drinks! LOL. As a fan of soft drinks it resulted in him not eating very healthy and gaining excessive weight over several years. His job at the time was with people who shared the mentality of eating whatever was fast and easy didn't help his situation. I found myself with a man who had become very unfit, overweight and suffering as a result of it. I, on the other-hand had always been a woman who had always prided herself in keeping fit and healthy and found this attitude of not caring about ones health or body very concerning and totally un-Islamic. Surely we owed it to ourselves to look after this God given amaanah (our body) in an intelligent fashion without succumbing to our desires (wants) of certain foods and drinks?

I realized that we cannot control others choices, albeit if they had chosen to not care so much about their health.

However, all of this was about to change. My husband and his younger brother booked a short trip away to South Korea. It was time for them to catch-up and spend some quality time together. Whilst travelling they decided to visit the DMZ (Demilitrisation Zone). They were very excited to visit the network of underground tunnels that were used during the war by the soldiers and spies. In they went like two little kids about to go on an adventure and out they came very soon after realizing how suffocating and tight it was down there, but not only that, my husband was struggling to climb out because of his weight, whilst also finding it hard to breathe. His brother was very upset to see him in this state and had a few harsh things to say to him, which brought my husband back to the reality that if he wanted energy with a healthy body he needed to make changes soon! This was the start of his weight loss journey. He approached me for my help and support and I was more than willing to lead the way.

After much research and using the knowledge of nutrition that I had gained whilst training for certain vocations over the years, I decided to switch to a healthy low carb keto diet which included throwing out all forms of sugar including fruits and adding lots of healthy fats including butter. YES, butter!

I learnt that the key to our bodies burning our own fat was to eat healthy fats! This may seem contradictory to some of you, but the food manufacturers from the past have drummed into us that a 'low fat, low calorie' diet is the key to losing weight and to keep away from all fats. That I can assure you is rubbish!

On the contrary most people felt starved and miserable whilst on those diets. I had been one of them in the distant past.

The KEY to burning fat was to keep our insulin level stable and this could only be done by pursuing a low carb keto lifestyle in combination with intermittent fasting (eating only during certain times of the day within a small window of time, example 8 hrs).

I became more and more creative in my cooking as I had to think out of the box, but we were really enjoying our food at the same time. My husband was dropping at least 1 kilo a week, sometimes 2, which kept us both motivated. After a while we found that we didn't want to eat any other way. I also incorporated monthly hijaamah detox sessions into my husband's new lifestyle plan which also helped to inspire eating healthy, because the last thing you want to do after a detox is to ruin the effects by loading your body with junk food!

Energy levels went up, lethargy went down, mental focus went up, aches & pains went out of the window and we both generally felt great! My husband lost around 20 kilos in the space of a few months, felt awesome and looked better than he ever had before. I must mention though that this was all done without any exercise! It just goes to show how food impacts our bodies. SubhaanAllaah.

As a result of changing the way we eat I also lost weight which I'm certainly not complaining about as I had also become a little overweight by indulging a little here and there, but in order not to lose too much weight I eventually added 'healthy sugars' such as fruits back into my diet.

There is too much bad information out there concerning weight loss, numerous fad diets and extreme exercise regimes, none of which are required in order to lose fat and note I say lose fat NOT lose weight, because many times all people do is lose water weight and muscle resulting in an emaciated looking new-self! This is not what we should be aiming for. A healthy version of a low carb/keto way of eating includes plenty of fresh vegetables, salads, healthy fats and good quality protein, making sure that we do not become deficient in any way. I'm certainly no doctor or nutritionist but based on research and experience with my husband and hijaamah clients I do believe that this is one of the healthiest ways of eating out there."

COMMON MISTAKES PEOPLE MAKE WHEN TRYING TO LOSE WEIGHT

Losing weight can seem very tough. Sometimes you feel like you are doing everything right, yet still not getting results. You may actually be hindering your progress by following misguided or outdated advice. Here are common mistakes people make when trying to lose weight:

Only Focusing on the Scale Weight

It is very common to feel like you are not losing weight fast enough, despite faithfully sticking to your diet. However, the number on the scale is only one measure of weight change. Weight is influenced by several things, including fluid fluctuations and how much food remains in your system. In fact, weight can fluctuate by up to 4 lbs (1.8 kg) over the course of a day, depending on how much food and liquid you have consumed. Also, increased estrogen levels and other hormonal changes in women can lead to greater water retention, which is reflected in scale weight. If the number on the scale isn't moving, you may very well be losing fat mass but holding on to water.

Fortunately, you can do several things to lose water weight. If you've been working out, you may be gaining muscle and losing fat. When this happens, your clothes may start to feel looser especially around the waist despite a stable scale weight. Measuring your waist with a tape measure can reveal you are actually losing fat, even if the scale number doesn't change much.

Bottom Line: Many factors can affect scale weight, including fluid fluctuations, muscle mass gain and the weight of undigested food. You may be losing body fat even if the scale reading doesn't change much.

Eating Too Many or Too Few Calories

A calorie deficit is required for weight loss. This means you need to burn more calories than you consume. For many years, it was believed that a decrease of 3,500 calories per week would result in 1 lb (.45 kg) of fat loss. However, recent research shows the calorie deficit needed varies from person to person. You may feel as though you are not eating very many calories; but in fact, most of us have a tendency to underestimate and under report what we eat.

In a two-week study, 10 obese people reported consuming 1,000 calories per day. Lab testing showed they were actually taking in about 2,000 calories per day. You may be consuming too many foods that are healthy but also high in calories, such as nuts and cheese. Watching portion sizes is key. On the other hand, decreasing your calorie intake too much can be counterproductive. Studies on very low-calorie diets providing less than 1,000 calories per day show they can lead to muscle loss and slow down metabolism significantly.

Bottom Line: Consuming too many calories can stop you from losing weight. On the other hand, too few calories can make you ravenously hungry and reduce your metabolism and muscle mass.

Not Exercising or Exercising Too Much

During weight loss, you inevitably lose some muscle mass as well as fat, although the amount depends on several factors. If you don't exercise at all while restricting calories, you're likely to lose more muscle mass and experience a decrease in metabolic rate. By contrast, exercising helps minimize the amount of lean mass you lose, boost fat loss and prevent your metabolism from slowing down. The more lean mass you have, the easier it is to lose weight and maintain the weight loss.

Over-exercising can also cause problems. Studies show excessive exercise is unsustainable in the long term for most people and may lead to stress. In addition, it may impair the production of adrenal hormones that regulate stress response. Trying to force your body to burn more calories by exercising too much is neither effective nor healthy. Lifting weights and doing cardio several times per week is a sustainable strategy for maintaining metabolic rate during weight loss.

Bottom Line: A lack of exercise can lead to loss of muscle mass and lower metabolism. On the other hand, too much exercise is neither healthy nor effective, and it may lead to severe stress if anything.

Not Lifting Weights

Performing resistance training is incredibly important during weight loss. Studies show lifting weights is one of the most effective exercise strategies for gaining muscle and increasing metabolic rate. It also improves overall body composition and boosts belly fat loss. In fact, a review of 15 studies with more than 700 people found the best strategy of all for weight loss appears to be combined aerobic exercise and weightlifting.

Bottom Line: Weightlifting or resistance training can help boost metabolic rate, increase muscle mass and promote fat loss, including belly fat.

Choosing Low-Fat or "Diet" Foods

Processed low-fat or "diet" foods are often considered good choices for losing weight, but they may actually have the opposite effect. Many of these products are loaded with sugar to improve their taste. For instance, one cup (245 grams) of low-fat, fruit-flavored yogurt can contain a whopping 47 grams of sugar (nearly 12 teaspoons). Rather than keep you full, low-fat products are likely to make you hungrier, so you end up eating even more. Instead of low-fat or "diet" foods, choose a combination of nutritious, minimally processed foods.

Bottom Line: Fat-free or "diet" foods are typically high in sugar and may lead to hunger and higher calorie intake.

Overestimating How Many Calories You Burn During Exercise

Many people believe that exercise "supercharges" their metabolism. Although exercise increases metabolic rate somewhat, it may actually be less than you think. Studies show both normal and overweight people tend to overestimate the number of calories they burn during exercise, often by a significant amount. In one study, people burned 200 and 300 calories during exercise sessions. Yet when asked, they estimated they had burned over 800 calories. As a result, they ended up eating more. That being said, exercise is still crucial for overall health and can help you lose weight. It is just not as effective at burning calories as some people think.

Bottom Line: Studies show people tend to overestimate the number of calories they burn during exercise.

Not Eating Enough Protein

Getting enough protein is extremely important if you are trying to lose weight. Protein has shown to help with weight loss in several ways. It can reduce appetite, increase feelings of fullness, decrease calorie intake, increase metabolic rate and protect muscle mass during weight loss. In a 12-day study, people ate a diet containing 30% of calories from protein. They ended up consuming an average of 575 fewer calories per day than when they ate 15% of calories from protein. A review also found that higher-protein diets, containing 0.6–0.8 grams of protein per pound (1.2–1.6 g/kg), may benefit appetite control and body composition. To optimize weight loss, make sure each of your meals contains a high-protein food.

Bottom Line: High protein intake helps with weight loss by reducing appetite, increasing feelings of fullness and boosting metabolic rate.

Not Eating Enough Fiber

A low-fiber diet may be compromising your weight loss efforts. Studies show a type of soluble fiber known as viscous fiber helps reduce appetite by forming a gel that holds water. This gel moves slowly through your digestive tract, making you feel full. Research suggests all types of fibers benefit weight loss. However, a review of several studies found viscous fiber reduced appetite and calorie intake much more than other types. When total fiber intake is high, some of the calories from foods in mixed meals aren't absorbed. Researchers estimate that doubling daily fiber intake could result in up to 130 fewer calories being absorbed.

Bottom Line: Eating enough fiber can help reduce appetite by filling you up so you eat less. It may also help you absorb fewer calories from other foods.

Eating Too Much Fat on a Low-Carb Diet

Ketogenic and low-carb diets can be very effective for weight loss. Studies show they tend to reduce appetite, which often leads to a spontaneous reduction in calorie intake. Many low-carb and ketogenic diets allow unlimited amounts of fat, assuming that the resulting appetite suppression will keep calories low enough for weight loss. However, some people may not experience a strong enough signal to stop eating. As a result, they may be consuming too many calories to achieve a calorie deficit. If you are adding large amounts of fat to your food or beverages and are not losing weight, you may want to cut back on the fat.

Bottom Line: Although low-carb and ketogenic diets help reduce hunger and calorie intake, adding too much fat may slow down or prevent weight loss.

Eating Too Often, Even If You Are Not Hungry

For many years, the conventional advice has been to eat every few hours in order to prevent hunger and experience a drop in metabolism. Unfortunately, this can lead to too many calories being consumed over the course of the day. You may also never truly feel full. In one study, blood sugar levels and hunger decreased while metabolic rate and feelings of fullness increased in men who consumed 3 meals versus 14 meals within a 36-hour time frame.

The recommendation to eat breakfast every morning, regardless of appetite, also appears to be misguided. One study found when people skipped breakfast, they took in more calories at lunch than when they had eaten a morning meal. However, overall they consumed an average of 408 fewer calories for the day. Eating when you are hungry and only when you are hungry seems to be the key to successful weight loss. However, letting yourself get too hungry is also a bad idea. It is better to eat a snack than become ravenously hungry, which can cause you to make poor food decisions.

Bottom Line: Eating too often can hurt your weight loss efforts. For the best results, it is important to eat only when you are hungry.

Having Unrealistic Expectations

Having weight loss and other health-related goals can help keep you motivated. But having unrealistic expectations can actually work against you. Researchers analyzed data from several weight loss center programs. They reported overweight and obese women who expected to lose the most weight were the most likely to drop out of a program after 6 to 12 months. Adjust your expectations to a more realistic and modest goal, such as a 10% drop in weight in one year. This can help prevent you from getting discouraged and improve your chances for success.

Bottom Line: Unrealistic expectations can lead to frustration and giving up altogether. Make your goals more modest to increase your chances of successful weight loss.

Not Tracking What You Eat In Any Way

Eating nutritious foods is a good weight loss strategy. However, you may still be eating more calories than you need to lose weight. What's more, you may not be getting the right amount of protein, fiber, carbohydrates and fat to support your weight loss efforts. Studies show that tracking what you eat can help you get an accurate picture of your calorie and nutrient consumption, as well as provide accountability. In addition to food, most online tracking sites and apps allow you to enter your daily exercise as well.

Bottom Line: If you are not tracking what you eat, you may be consuming more calories than you realize. You may also be getting less protein and fiber than you think.

Still Drinking Sugar

Many people cut soft drinks and other sweetened beverages out of their diet to lose weight, which is a good thing. However, drinking fruit juice instead isn't smart. Even 100% fruit juice is loaded with sugar and may lead to health and weight problems similar to those caused by sugar-sweetened beverages. For instance, 12 ounces (320 grams) of unsweetened apple juice contain 36 grams of sugar. That's even more than in 12 ounces of cola. What's more, liquid calories don't seem to affect the appetite centers in your brain the same way calories from solid foods do. Studies show that you end up consuming more calories overall, instead of compensating for the liquid calories by eating less later in the day.

Bottom Line: If you cut out sugar-sweetened beverages but continue drinking fruit juice, you are still getting a lot of sugar and are likely to take in more calories overall.

Not Reading Labels

Failing to accurately read label information can cause you to consume unwanted calories and unhealthy ingredients. Unfortunately, many foods are labeled with healthy-sounding food claims on the front of the package. These may give you a false sense of security about choosing a certain item. To get to the most important information for weight control, you need to look at the ingredients list and nutrition facts label, which are on the back of the container.

Bottom Line: Food labels provide information on ingredients, calories and nutrients. Make sure you understand how to accurately read labels.

CHAPTER TWELVE

NEVER GIVE UP ON LOSING WEIGHT

We experience a lot in life. We gain weight when we get pregnant, when we are under a lot of stress, when we are celebrating a special occasion, when we are vacationing, when we are in grief, etc. There are many reasons we women gain weight, and it is okay. It is okay to gain a few pounds under certain circumstances because that is what life is all about. However, we should be mindful about it, and have a plan to lose it after. We should give ourselves 5-10 pounds and then a plan to lose it if we go above that.

I know that you are busy. I know that you are juggling many hats; between being a mom, a cook, a janitor, a wife, a daughter, a driver, having a job, a student, etc. However, with just a few small changes in your life you will be able to lose weight while juggling all of that. Losing weight is 80% about the foods we eat and 20% exercise. As moms we move a lot and are burning calories here and there.

Losing weight is a tough path to take. There's plenty standing in your way - societal pressures, a sedentary lifestyle, a lazy metabolism, hunger pangs ... and then when you go to the gym, all those flat-bellied women stare at you as if your gut's hanging halfway down to your knees. It is easy to think about giving up when faced with all of these obstacles.

In today's fast paced life the need for effective fat loss is considered essential in order to maintain good health. While fat loss has often been linked to those who are obese, it is also considered suitable for those who are slightly overweight. Fat loss does not involve spending thousands of dollars and can be achieved if you know the tricks of the trade.

In shaa' Allaah this book has covered those tricks and has opened your eyes to a new way to eat and live. As a Muslim woman our motivation is to please Allaah from every angle. By being healthy and active this is something that Allaah will be pleased with in shaa' Allaah. By being healthy and active we are able to be better servants to our Lord. We can do more ibaadah, we can help more people, we can achieve more goals in shaa' Allaah. We need to remember this intention the entire time and work to achieve the goals we set for our weight for the sake of Allaah. It is not just about looking nice in our abaayahs, it's more about how we feel when we get up to pray, to play with our kids, to complete the jobs we have to complete daily in shaa' Allaah.

May Allaah allow us to be those believers who He is pleased with - Aameen.

Have you bought "SuperCharge Homeschooling's The Power of Reading Curriculum"

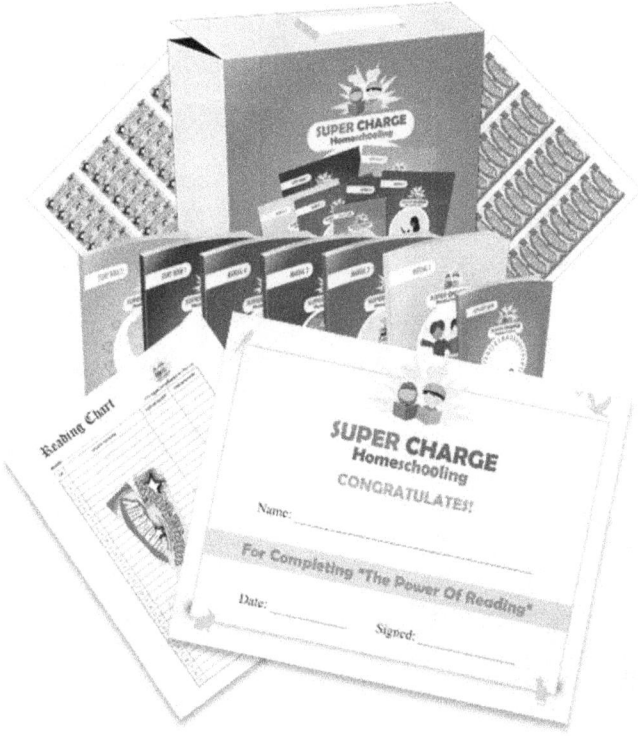

Have you bought "SuperCharge Homeschooling's Pre-K & Kindergarten Curriculum"

Pre-K Curriculum

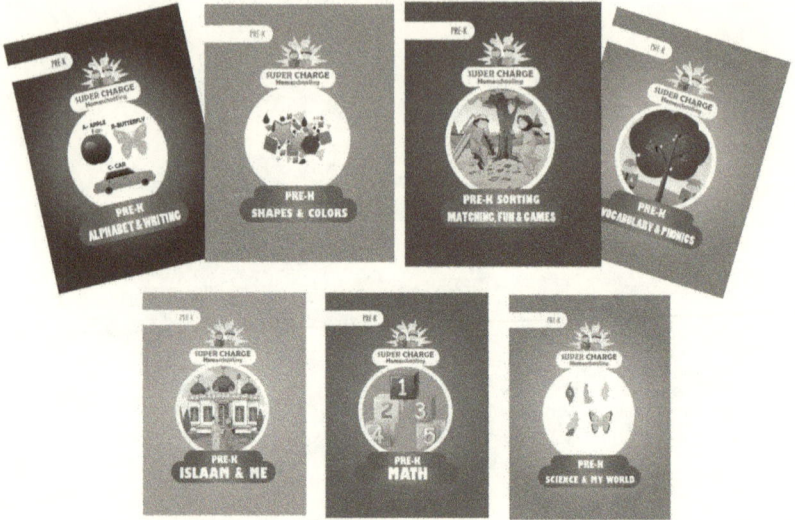

Kindergarten Curriculum

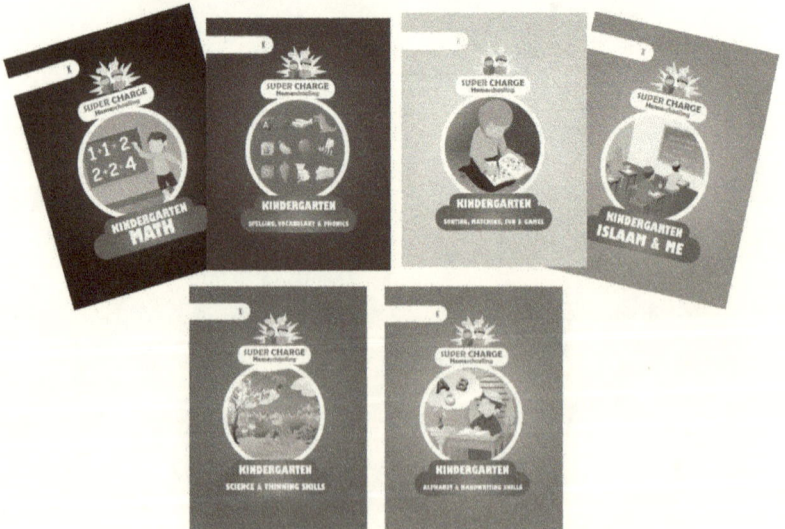

Have You Bought The Series: "Things Every Kid Should Know: Drugs, Alcohol, Smoking, Bullying, Junk Food and Amr's Adventure in Europe" for Your Kids By Alya Nuri?

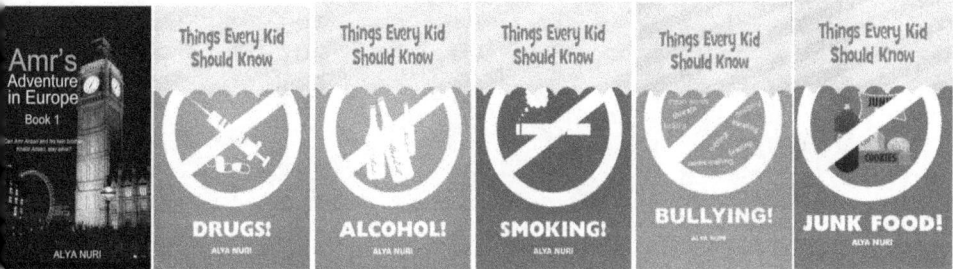

Have You Bought The Series: "Things Every Kid Should Know: Strangers, Reduce, Re-use & Recycle, Fire and Muslim Boys" for Your Kids By Zafar Nuri?

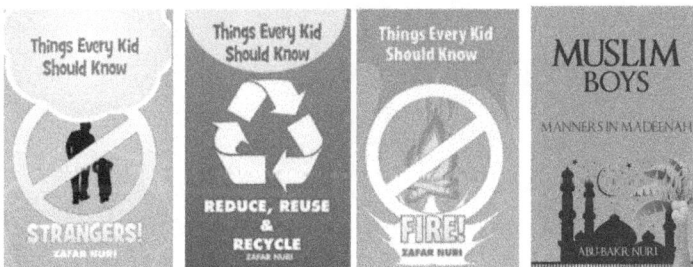

Have You Bought The Series: "Things Every Kid Should Know: Hand Washing, Teeth, Stealing and Cheating" for Your Kids By Arsalon Nuri?

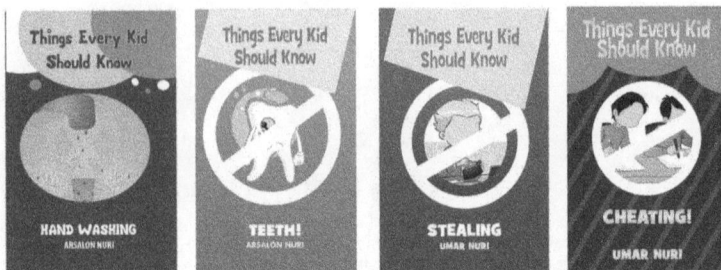

Have You Bought The Series: "Things Every Kid Should Know: Obeying Parents!" for Your Kids By Asiya Nuri?

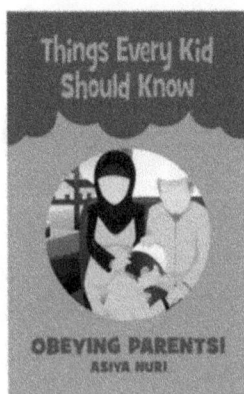

Books By Zohra Sarwari

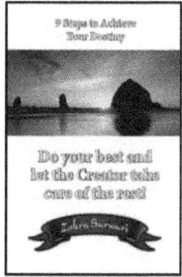

9 Steps to Achieve Your Destiny

Do your best and let the Creator take care of the rest!

Zohra Sarwari

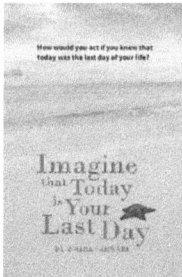

How would you act if you knew that today was the last day of your life?

Imagine that Today is Your Last Day

BY: ZOHRA SARWARI

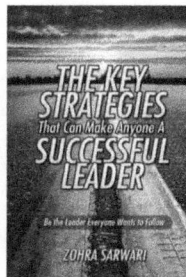

THE KEY STRATEGIES That Can Make Anyone A SUCCESSFUL LEADER

Be the Leader Everyone Wants to Follow

ZOHRA SARWARI

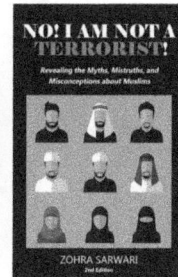

NO! I AM NOT A TERRORIST!

Revealing the Myths, Mistruths, and Misconceptions about Muslims

ZOHRA SARWARI
2nd Edition

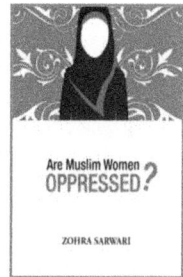

Are Muslim Women OPPRESSED?

ZOHRA SARWARI

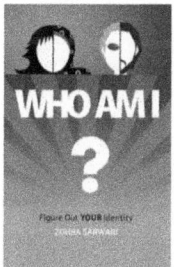

WHO AM I ?

Figure Out YOUR Identity

ZOHRA SARWARI

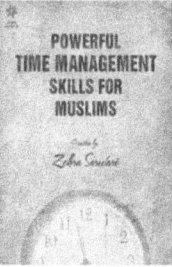

POWERFUL TIME MANAGEMENT SKILLS FOR MUSLIMS

Zohra Sarwari

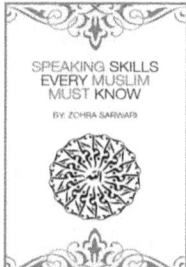

SPEAKING SKILLS EVERY MUSLIM MUST KNOW

BY: ZOHRA SARWARI

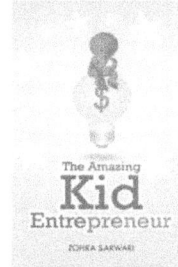

The Amazing Kid Entrepreneur

ZOHRA SARWARI

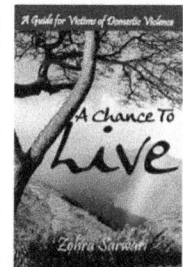

A Guide for Victims of Domestic Violence

A Chance To Live

Zohra Sarwari

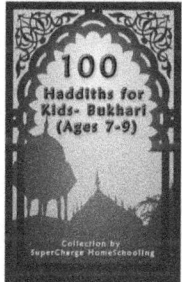

100 Haddiths for Kids- Bukhari (Ages 7-9)

Collection by SuperCharge HomeSchooling

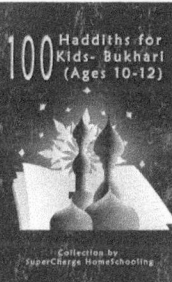

100 Haddiths for Kids- Bukhari (Ages 10-12)

Collection by SuperCharge HomeSchooling

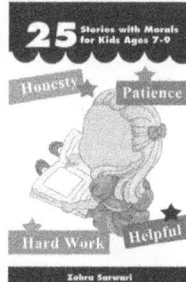

25 Stories with Morals for Kids Ages 7-9

Honesty Patience

Hard Work Helpful

Zohra Sarwari

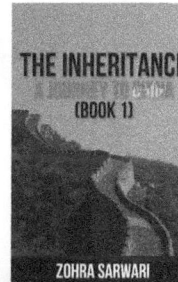

THE INHERITANCE A JOURNEY TO AFRICA (BOOK 1)

ZOHRA SARWARI

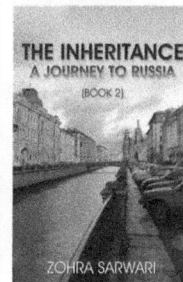

THE INHERITANCE A JOURNEY TO RUSSIA (BOOK 2)

ZOHRA SARWARI

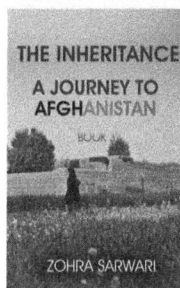

THE INHERITANCE A JOURNEY TO AFGHANISTAN BOOK

ZOHRA SARWARI

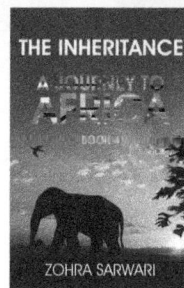

THE INHERITANCE A JOURNEY TO AFRICA BOOK 4

ZOHRA SARWARI

Books by Zohra Sarwari

www.ingramcontent.com/pod-product-compliance
Lightning Source LLC
Chambersburg PA
CBHW030025290326
41934CB00005B/490